TOTAL
TAI CHI

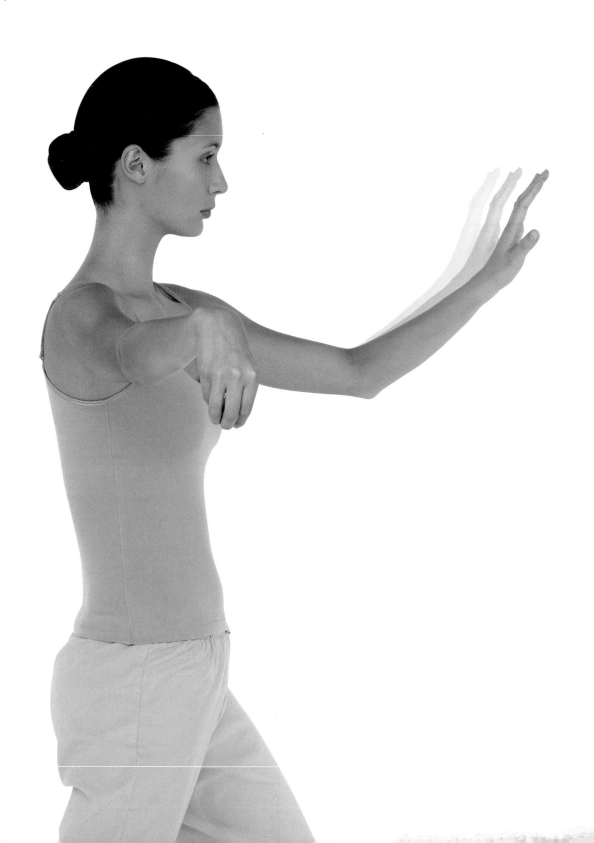

TOTAL
TAI CHI

*The step-by-step guide
to Tai Chi at home
for everybody*

RONNIE ROBINSON

DUNCAN BAIRD PUBLISHERS

LONDON

Total Tai Chi
Ronnie Robinson

Distributed in the USA and Canada by
Sterling Publishing Co., Inc.
387 Park Avenue South
New York, NY 10016-8810

This revised edition first published in the UK and USA in 2009 by
Duncan Baird Publishers Ltd
Sixth Floor, Castle House
75–76 Wells Street
London W1T 3QH

Managing Editor: Grace Cheetham
Editor: Kesta Desmond
Managing Designer: Daniel Sturges
Picture Research: Louise Glasson
Commissioned photography: Matthew Ward

Library of Congress Cataloging-in-Publication Data

Robinson, Ronnie.
  Total tai-chi : the step-by-step guide to tai chi at home for
everybody / Ronnie Robinson.
    p. cm.
  Includes index.
  ISBN 978-1-84483-723-6
  1. Tai chi. I. Title.
  GV504.R62 2009
  796.815'5--dc22

                                    2008018754

10 9 8 7 6 5 4 3 2 1

Typeset in Trade Gothic
Color reproduction by Scanhouse, Malaysia
Printed in Singapore by Imago

Publisher's note:
Before following any advice or practice suggested in this book,
it is recommended that you consult your doctor as to its
suitability, especially if you suffer from any health problems
or special conditions. The publishers, the author, and the
photographers cannot accept responsibility for any injuries or
damage incurred as a result of following the exercises in this
book, or of using any of the therapeutic methods described or
mentioned here.

For information about custom editions, special sales,
premium and corporate purchases, please contact
Sterling Special Sales Department at 800-805-5489 or
specialsales@sterlingpub.com.

"The water of the spring is clear, like fine crystal.

The water of the pond lies still and placid.

Your mind should be as the water and your

spirit like the spring."

THE EIGHT TRUTHS OF TAI CHI

contents

how to use this book

Everyone can learn the art of tai chi. No special equipment is required and you can train almost anywhere and at any time. Before you start, it can help to know something about the underlying principles of tai chi, its history and styles, and what the benefits are. You will find this information in Chapter 1. Then, in Chapter 2, I describe some of the practical principles that will guide you in tai chi. For example, the importance of being grounded so that your weight and energy are centred in your lower body while your upper body remains light and free.

Chapter 3 consists of a series of warm-up exercises. Some of them are standard warm-ups that you might do prior to any type of exercise. Others are from the Chinese art of chi kung (see pages 26–7) and are specifically designed to get chi flowing through your meridians in preparation for your tai chi practice.

The photographs and captions in Chapter 4 guide you through the movements of the tai chi Hand Form. Although the practice of tai chi is, ultimately, about identifying and aligning yourself with the simplicity of the work, the act of learning the postures can often seem difficult. Study the photographs carefully, and allow plenty of time for the information to transfer from your brain to your body – ultimately, the movements will become reflexive, but don't expect this to happen overnight. Most people who view a performance of tai chi are struck by its grace and beauty. What makes it so aesthetically pleasing is that there are no extraneous movements, no over-extending, nothing to jar the eye – just pure simplicity. Everything is exactly where it needs to be. Ergonomically, tai chi is about completing an action in the optimum way. When learning and practising, try to remind yourself of the basic simplicity of tai chi.

Chapter 5 shows you how to do tai chi with a partner. These exercises will help you to deepen your understanding of tai chi and give you a tool with which to evaluate your performance.

The final chapter of the book is about meditation – how to reach a place of mental stillness. Try the different techniques I describe and see which ones work best for you. The book closes with a short section in which I suggest ways in which you can reflect upon on your practice.

Whether you are a complete beginner, or have studied tai chi for some time, there is much within this book to inspire you or deepen your level of practice. Go slowly forward with a calm, open mind, a relaxed body and a patient heart and you will discover many things that will improve your mental, physical and spiritual well-being. The art of tai chi has the potential to reach far beyond a simple physical exercise. Let it become an integral part of the way you walk, breathe, think and relate to everything that is involved in 21st-century living.

grids, symbols and arrows

THE FOOT GRIDS AND ARROWS IN CHAPTERS 3, 4 and 5

The positioning of your feet – and of your body in relation to your feet – is important in tai chi (and also when you are warming up for tai chi; see Chapter 3). To help you position yourself as accurately as possible, I have included grids to show you where to place your feet and body in each movement. Try to get your feet to match the direction, angle (of one foot to the other) and spacing of the blue footprints in each grid. Your body should face the same way and be in the same position (relative to your feet) as the brown line. In Chapter 5 the diagrams are expanded to show the correct positioning of your partner's feet

and body as well as yours. In addition to the foot grids, I have included arrows on some of the photographs in chapters 3, 4 and 5. These indicate the direction in which you should be moving, pushing or turning.

SYMBOLS USED IN THIS BOOK

👁 A visualization that helps to focus your mind.

💡 A practical tip, idea or comment.

❋ Advice about how to breathe.

★ A word of caution.

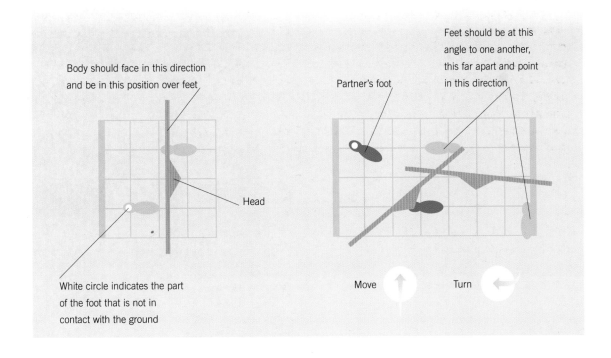

Body should face in this direction and be in this position over feet

Head

White circle indicates the part of the foot that is not in contact with the ground

Partner's foot

Feet should be at this angle to one another, this far apart and point in this direction

Move   Turn

introduction

When I was at school, I had very little interest in sports such as football, cricket or running. Later, when I approached my mid-20s, I developed an interest in personal development that led me to try meditation. However, at that point in time, my mind was too busy for me to sit quietly in contemplation. I soon became frustrated by my inability to sit still for any length of time. I knew there were many benefits to be gained from meditation, but I just couldn't settle down.

In retrospect, I realize that what I needed was something that would occupy my busy mind while simultaneously quietening me down. I was searching for something that contained elements of active participation and passive introspection. By accident, or perhaps by greater design, I picked up some information on a new tai chi class for beginners. Because tai chi was relatively new in Western terms, there were very few trained teachers around. The person who led our class had attended a weekend seminar and guided us through what basics he could remember. We spent a couple of hours slowly and quietly walking across the floor, focusing on being relaxed and quiet, and paying close attention to each and every step. For some reason I liked it enough to go back the following week. From these first lessons I have continued tai chi and have tried to integrate the art into every aspect of my life.

I have practised tai chi for nearly quarter of a century and it has had a profound effect on me. On a simple level it has helped me to achieve a very deep sense of my body and how I use – or abuse – it. My practice acts as a daily checklist of where I am with my body, with my inner self and in relationship to others. I firmly believe that, through the practice of tai chi, I have developed a deeper understanding of the physical, mental and emotional aspects of not only my own being, but also that of others. This enables me to act in a clearer, more focused manner, from a position of inner strength. I have also found a way to be quiet when necessary and to be aware of when my mind gets too busy.

In Western terms, tai chi was virtually unknown 50 years ago whereas now it is not only widely accepted but also greatly enjoyed by hundreds of thousands of practitioners. It is now taught and practised in health centres, hospitals, offices, prisons, schools, universities, health clubs, stress centres, centres for the elderly and martial art clubs.

Having taught tai chi in a wide range of environments, I have also experienced the many benefits this art can have on students of all ages and physical abilities. These benefits range from feeling healthier and more alive, to discovering what it is that you really want to achieve from your life. Tai chi is a truly multi-faceted art that offers many things to many people. Within these pages, I hope to provide you with simple, yet practical guidance to help you to make the first steps on your tai chi journey.

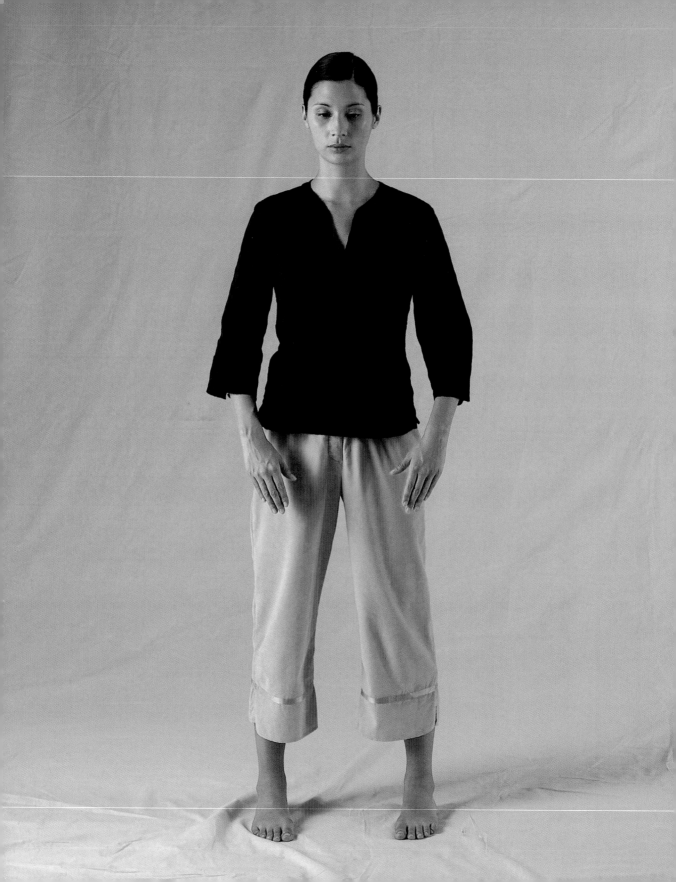

introducing tai chi

Tai chi is a Chinese exercise system that, through the practice of gentle, flowing movements, trains the body to move in the very best way it can, and simultaneously calms the mind. Rooted in principles from 4,000 years ago, this ancient art is now practised throughout the world by people of all ages and levels of physical fitness.

In this chapter, I introduce some of the underlying principles of the art, such as yin and yang, and chi (internal energy). I also trace the history of tai chi from its reputed origin on the holy Taoist mountain of Wudang Shan through to today's proliferation of tai chi styles.

what is tai chi?

Tai chi is an ancient martial art that was once performed by reclusive, devoted Taoist monks on Wudang Mountain in China. Today, it is practised in a wide variety of places from dedicated tai chi classes in martial art schools to predominantly health-related classes in health centres and hospitals in city centres all over the world. Since its early beginnings, there have been a number of changes in the way that tai chi is taught and there are now a plethora of styles. What is common to most forms of tai chi is the benefits they offer in terms of health, posture, confidence, mental focus and spiritual development.

Tai chi is part of the Chinese tradition of chi kung, which is a system of exercises that encourage chi energy (see pages 24–7) to flow freely around the body. Today, the term tai chi is applied to an incredible number of interpretations of the original Chinese martial art. Essentially, tai chi is a series of postures, known as the Hand Form (see pages 48–9), that are performed in a smooth, flowing manner over a period of time ranging from 3 to 20 minutes, depending on the style of tai chi (see pages 20–23). The postures, which were inspired by the fluid movement of various creatures, were originally used for self-defence. In addition to the Hand Form, there are also Weapon Forms of tai chi.

Supreme ultimate fist

The words "tai chi" can be translated as "supreme ultimate". And the full name given to the art – "tai chi chuan" – can be translated as "supreme ultimate fist" or "supreme ultimate boxing". Tai chi chuan is a system of fighting that is based on applying the inter-relationship of yin and yang.

Although tai chi was once used for self-defence, it is not often used for this purpose today. But the principles of tai chi still serve us well because we can apply them to psychological or emotional as well as physical attack. On a basic level, if any type of force (yang) comes toward you, it should be met with softness (yin).

Yin and yang

Tai chi is symbolically represented by the image of yin and yang. Yin and yang are two complementary yet opposing forces that together make up "the whole". Yin is characterized by softness, darkness, coldness and passivity. Yang is characterized by hardness, light, heat and action. Neither yin nor yang is superior to the other – instead, they complement each other perfectly.

The yin yang symbol is used to illustrate many aspects of Chinese health and culture in practices ranging from Traditional Chinese Medicine and acupuncture to Chinese geomancy or feng shui. The qualities of yin and yang symbolize all that is present in the universe.

The white side of the yin yang symbol is the yang aspect and the black side is the yin aspect. The white side contains a black spot and the black side contains a white spot – this symbolizes the idea that yin and yang always contain an aspect of each other; that nothing is totally black or white. Imagine, for example, how stars shine on the darkest night or how, on the brightest day, there are shadows.

RIGHT: Every morning people practise tai chi in outdoor spaces all over China. This ancient martial art is characterized by its sequence of beautiful, slow and fluid movements.

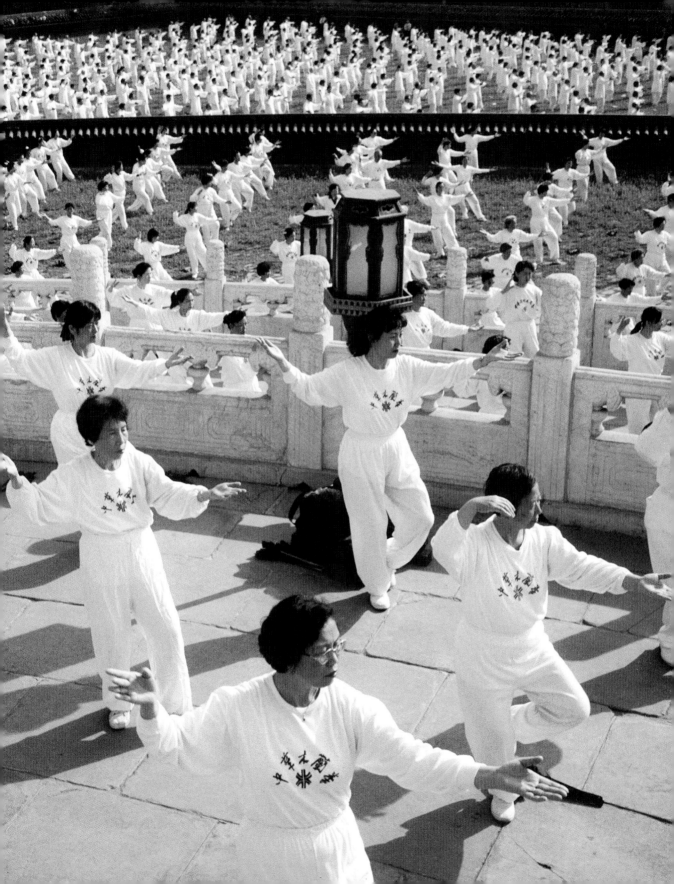

The characteristics of yin and yang

The concepts of yin and yang help us to understand that all things must be understood in relation to one another. We define things in relation to their opposites. For example, we couldn't measure hot if we didn't have cold, and we couldn't define night if there were no such thing as day. The entire universe is divided into opposites: that which is yin and that which is yang.

Yang	Yin
Sun	Moon
Day	Night
Male	Female
Summer	Winter
Hot	Cold
Hard	Soft
Outside	Inside
Active	Passive
Motion	Stillness
Light	Shade

Applying yin and yang in tai chi

Understanding the interplay of yin and yang is fundamental to tai chi practice. For example, if you push your arms out in front of you as far as you can, while leaning forward until your back leg is locked, your body will be in extreme yang. It wouldn't take much force to push or pull you off balance. If, however, you stand with your elbows bent, your knees soft and your shoulders relaxed, you will have a better balance between the aspects of yin and yang. This means that you will be more able to maintain your central equilibrium and move in the most efficient way possible.

Imagine that you are under attack from an opponent during tai chi. If you greet a strong force with a strong defence, you are greeting a yang action with a yang response. This creates the potential for damage. For example, if you raise your arm to block a punch to your head, the combination of two hard forces may hurt both you and your attacker. If, on the other hand, you meet a yang force with a yin force, by, for example, moving slightly and making contact with your opponent's fist softly from the side, you may be able to evade and neutralize the attack.

TAI CHI COMES FROM WU CHI

In Chinese philosophy, tai chi comes from Wu Chi. According to ancient Chinese belief, Wu Chi is the void or state of emptiness that existed before creation. It is usually depicted pictorially as an empty circle. Out of the void (Wu Chi) comes action (tai chi). In practical terms, you can think of Wu Chi as the state of emptiness or clarity that you seek before you begin your tai chi practice.

The relationship between tai chi and Wu Chi can be described like this: "Tai chi [supreme ultimate] emanates from the Wu Chi [void] and is the mother of yin and yang. In movement tai chi separates. In stillness yin and yang blend and return to Wu Chi." (Wang Tsung Yueh, 18th century.)

The following analogy also helps to explain the relationship between Wu Chi and tai chi: picture a school gym in the early hours of the morning. No one is in it – it is completely empty – there is no one even to acknowledge its existence. Therefore, the gym has no "meaning". This is the state of Wu Chi. Now imagine the doors of the gym opening in the morning and a group of children running in. Suddenly there is activity in the room – the room has a sense of meaning and being. This is the state of tai chi.

THE TEXTS OF TAI CHI

The texts of tai chi are known collectively as the *Tai Chi Classics*. Although the bulk of the texts (including the passage below) have been credited to Wang Tsung Yueh (18th century), there are a number of other authors whose exact identities remain unclear.

THE TREATISE ON TAI CHI CHUAN

Tai chi [supreme ultimate] emanates from the Wu Chi [void] and is the mother of yin and yang.

In movement tai chi separates.

In stillness yin and yang blend and return to Wu Chi.

It is not deficient or excessive.

It adheres to an extension and follows a bend.

I remain soft when my opponent is hard, this is called yielding.

When I follow my opponent he becomes backed up; this is called adherence.

If my opponent's movement is fast,

Then I respond quickly.

When his movement is slow,

Then I follow slowly.

Although there are countless variations, the principles that pervade remain the same.

By being familiar with his touch, one gradually understands *chin* [intrinsic strength].

In understanding *chin* one can attain wisdom.

Without continued practice, one will have difficulties in understanding tai chi.

Without undue effort, the chin reaches the headtop.

Allow the chi [vital energy] to sink to the dantien [elixir field].

Don't incline in any direction.

Suddenly appear.

Suddenly disappear.

When force comes to the left, empty that side; and do similar when force is at the right.

When the opponent rises up, I appear taller; when he sinks down, then I sink lower.

In advancing, he finds my distance too long.

In retreating, my distance is frustratingly short.

A feather cannot be placed, and a fly cannot land on any part of my body.

My opponent cannot know me, but I alone know him.

Becoming an unequalled boxer is a result of this.

There are many fighting arts.

And although they use other forms, in the main, they never go beyond the strong overcoming the weak, and the slow losing to the fast.

The strong overcoming the weak and the slow losing to the fast are all the result of natural abilities and not well-trained techniques.

From the saying, "A thousand pounds can be deflected by four ounces", we understand that this technique is not a result of using strength.

An old person who can defeat a group of young people – how can this be due to speed?

Stand like a perfectly balanced scale and move like a rotating wheel.

Sinking to one side creates flowing movement; being double-weighted is sluggish.

One who has spent years of practice and still can't neutralize, and is always controlled by his opponent; he has not overcome the fault of double-weightedness.

To overcome this fault one must distinguish yin and yang.

Adherence means yielding and yielding means adherence.

Inside yin there is yang.

Inside yang there is yin.

Yin and yang mutually assist and change each other.

In understanding this you will understand *chin*.

Once you understand *chin*, and the more you practice, the more skill you will develop.

Quietly respect knowledge and turn it over in your mind.

Gradually you will do as you wish.

Basically, it's giving up yourself to follow others.

Most people erroneously give up the close to find the far.

It is said, "Missing it by a mile will take you many miles astray." The practitioner must carefully study.

This is the Treatise.

the origins of tai chi

Legend has it that tai chi originated on Wudang Shan, a sacred mountain in China, with a man called Chang San Feng. Although it is accepted that Chang San Feng existed, there is much debate about how tai chi developed after him and even whether he is its legitimate creator.

Chang San Feng

According to legend, Chan San Feng (1279–1368) was a government official who retired from working life in order to further his spiritual development. He went to live in harmony with nature in a secluded cave on Wudang Shan mountain in northwest Hubei Province. He spent the remainder of his life here in deep contemplation.

One day, during his regular meditation, Chang San Feng is said to have dreamed or visualized a fight between a snake and a crane. Whenever the snake hissed at the bird, the bird would raise its wings and retreat. Similarly, as the bird dipped down to attack the snake with its beak, the snake would slither out of reach. In Chang's dream, the fight went on for some time, but neither creature was harmed or defeated.

TAI CHI AND TAOISM

Many of the principles of tai chi originate from the ancient Chinese philosophy of Taoism, which is concerned with achieving harmony with our environment and letting nature take its own course. The qualities of yielding, softness, slowness, balance and rootedness are central to both Taoism and tai chi.

The classic Taoist text *Tao Te Ching* (Way of Virtue) contains many of the ideas that lie at the heart of tai chi. It was reputedly written by the famous philosopher Lao Tzu. In the *Tao Te Ching*, Lao Tzu uses the image of a plant bending in the wind to explain how it is possible to yield to oncoming force (a core principle of tai chi). Bamboo is a plant that is prevalent in China and one can imagine Lao Tzu watching it blowing in a strong wind without breaking or snapping. It is this ability to stay rooted yet flexible in the face of adversity that makes tai chi effective and relevant, not just hundreds of years ago, but also in today's increasingly stressful

society. Some quotations from the *Tao Te Ching* that relate directly to tai chi are:

"Yield and overcome,
Bend and be straight."

And:

"Whosoever stands on tiptoe
does not stand firmly,
Whosoever stands with legs astride
will not advance."

The idea of using softness or yielding to overcome force makes tai chi into what the Chinese call an "internal" martial art. Other internal martial arts include Ba Gua Chuan and Hsing-I Chuan. Instead of using physical strength and force, these martial arts rely on the internal power of the practitioner. They are different from "external" martial art practices in that they don't depend on the strong overcoming the weak.

From this dream, Chang San Feng was inspired to create a system of self-defence that incorporated the natural movements of the snake and the bird, and other creatures. Chang is widely credited with creating a sequence of 13 martial art postures that went on to become tai chi. Among the movements he is credited with are White Crane Spreads Wings and Snake Creeps Down.

Many people would consider monks, such as Chang San Feng, to be peace-loving people who have no reason for learning martial combat techniques. However, in Cheng San Feng's time, the passivity of people living a contemplative life meant that they became easy prey for people who wanted to steal from them. Monks therefore needed a system of self-defence that relied upon defensive rather than offensive techniques.

Today, Wudang Shan is recognized as a World Heritage Site. It is a revered area in many ways. As well as being seen as an intensely spiritual place, 70 per cent of the herbs of the *Materia Medica*, the official bible of Traditional Chinese Medicine, grow on the mountain. Throughout history, holy Taoist monks have chosen to devote years to living in contemplation on these sacred peaks.

Contemporary theories

Although Chang San Feng was, for many years, credited as being the creator of the movements that became tai chi, contemporary historians tend to dispute this legend. They believe that the real home of tai chi may lie with the Chen family in Chenjiagou Village in China (see pages 20–21). Nevertheless, statues of Chang San Feng still exist in the temples of Wudang Shan, as does the cave that he is reputed to have inhabited. Many dedicated tai chi practitioners around the world continue to recognize Chang San Feng as the founder of the art.

BELOW: The mountain of Wudang Shan is reputed to be the birthplace of tai chi. Thousands of people visit it every year to pay homage to tai chi's legendary creator, Chang San Feng.

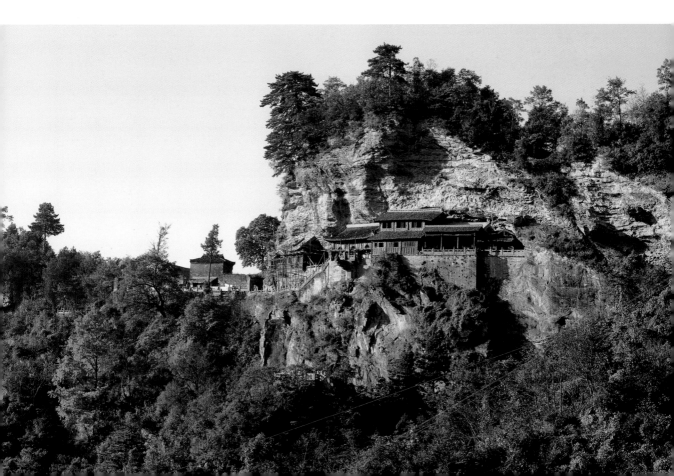

family styles of tai chi

Much of the very early history of tai chi is shrouded in mystery, but from the 17th century there is reliable written evidence to show that the art was being practised by the Chen family in China. For a long time the movements were a closely guarded family secret but, eventually, an outsider, Yang Lu Chan, gained access to them. From this point, tai chi skills began to spread and were passed down through the generations of several key families in China.

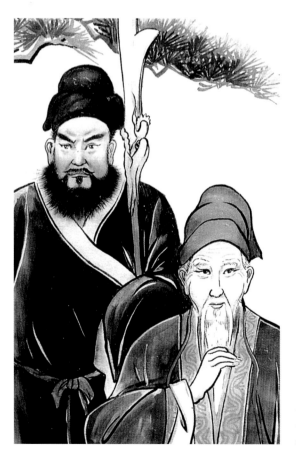

There are five major styles of tai chi: Chen, Yang, Wu (Hao), Wu and Sun. Each style is named after the Chinese family that taught – and still teaches – it. The Chen style of tai chi is the oldest and the Sun style is the most recent.

Chen style

According to reliable historical records, tai chi was being practised more than 300 years ago in China, in a place known as Chenjiagou (Chen) Village, Henan Province. Chen Wangting (1600–1680) created the first recognized system of the art by bringing together the various skills of Shaolin boxing, Traditional Chinese Medicine, chi kung breathing exercises, and the philosophical concepts of tai chi. Chen Wangting is thought to have begun teaching around 1650.

In Chen Wangting's time, it was considered very important to keep fighting skills within the family. This helped to provide the family members with a reasonable standard of living through regular work as fighters or bodyguards. Traditionally, only the men in the family were taught martial skills. It wasn't thought to be correct etiquette to teach women, and there was the additional danger that the skills would leak out when women left the family unit to get married.

LEFT: The original masters of tai chi were the male members of the Chen family in China. Tai chi was an important fighting skill and it was taught only to other family members.

To many of today's tai chi practitioners, the Chen style may appear strange. In contrast, to the slow, fluid movements usually associated with tai chi, Chen style tai chi is characterized by its sudden changes from fast to slow, stomping on the floor and rapid, explosive fist movements accompanied by loud shouts or roars. Anyone witnessing a performance of Chen style tai chi would have little doubt about its effectiveness as a martial art.

Since its early beginnings, Chen style tai chi has passed down through 16 generations of the family. Modern inheritors of the art include Chen Xiao Wang, Chen Zhenglei and Wang Haijun. They now teach regularly in Asia, Europe and America. Today, Chenjiagou Village is a popular tourist destination and many people go there to attend tai chi courses taught by the family members. It is also possible to attend or compete in an annual international tai chi competition held in Chenjiagou Village.

For many years the Chen family refused to teach outsiders, but eventually, in the 19th century, they trained a man called Yang Lu Chan who subsequently created the Yang style (see below). This break in the family tradition ultimately spawned other styles of tai chi too.

Yang style

Yang Lu Chan (1799–1872) is the person who is considered to be responsible for the spread of tai chi and the diversification of its styles. He entered the Chen family and, against the odds (given the great secrecy surrounding the family methods), he learned the art of tai chi.

Yang Lu Chan was born in Yongnian County in Hebei Province. In his youth he studied Shaolin boxing and developed a keen interest in martial arts. Yang heard about the effectiveness of Chen-style tai chi as a martial art and travelled to Chenjiagou Village in order to learn the system from the Chen family. However, as he was not part of the family, they refused to teach him their precious art. Legend has it that Yang succeeded in gaining employment as a servant in the Chen household in order secretly to learn the family art. As the Chen family members were conducting their daily training routine, Yang picked up the skills by quietly observing them. Then fate intervened to give him a helping hand.

One day, when all the men from the Chen family left the village, raiders came to rob the family. Yang Lu Chan was able to

TAI CHI DURING THE CULTURAL REVOLUTION

There was a point during the Cultural Revolution in China when the Chen style of tai chi was in danger of being lost forever. Because family units were contrary to the Communist ideal, many family-based activities were prohibited. For example, people were forced to destroy all their personal cooking utensils, not only to supply metal for arms, but also to destroy the family bonds that form through eating together. Tai chi was a cause of great concern to the authorities because it was practised within – and confined to – family units. In an interview I conducted with one of the Chen family members, Chen Zhenglei, he related a tale of how the Red Army broke his uncle's legs and dumped him in a well in order to prevent him teaching the family art. Other members of the family had to train in secret in order to keep the tradition alive. They even changed the names of some movements to make them more politically acceptable. For example, "Buddha Pounds the Mortar" was changed to "Pounding the Mortar for Mao".

apply his secretly acquired tai chi skills and successfully beat off the raiders. When the Chen elders returned and heard the story of Yang Lu Chan's heroic attack, they rewarded him with formal training in their family system.

Although this may be the stuff of legend, it is true that Yang went on to become highly skilled in tai chi and he helped to train the Emperor's army at the Imperial Palace in Beijing. Had it not been for Yang's travels beyond Chenjiagou Village, the art of tai chi may not have spread across China and, eventually, across the whole of the world.

Another factor that contributed to the spread of tai chi was the adaptations that Yang Lu Chuan made to the traditional Chen style. He removed many of the stomps and rapid punches, and this helped to make the Yang style of tai chi easier and more

BELOW: This tai chi practitioner moves slowly through the graceful dance-like movements of the Hand Form (Wu style). Not all styles of tai chi are slow and fluid. The original Chen style was known for its rapid fist movements and foot stomps.

accessible. The Yang style is characterized by open, expansive movements and, today, is probably the most popular type of tai chi that is practised.

Yang Chen Fu

Yang Lu Chuan passed his system of tai chi down through the generations. His grandson Yang Chen Fu (1883–1936) made a notable contribution to the spread of, not just Yang-style tai chi, but tai chi in general. He was invited by the Beijing Sports Society to teach tai chi in the city and he later travelled to other parts of China to teach Yang-style tai chi. He modified his grandfather's style, which made it significantly easier to learn, and helped to spread the art across China and make it a part of everyday life. In addition, Yang Chen Fu presented tai chi not just as a martial art but as a means of promoting health and well-being.

Yang Chen Fu was also responsible for producing some of the earliest written material on tai chi. Until that point many traditional tai chi practitioners were fighters who, in the main, were unable to read or write.

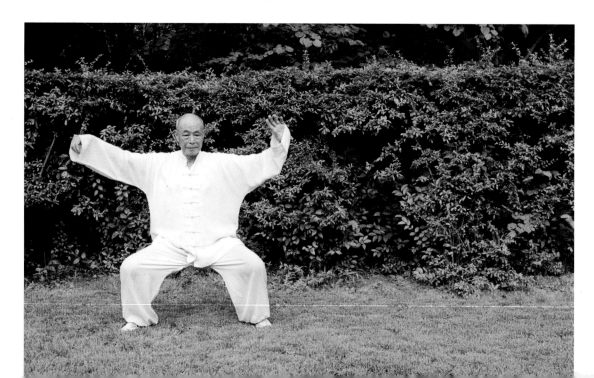

MANY DIFFERENT STYLES

In addition to the five family styles of tai chi described on pages 20–23, there are also a number of other recognized or accepted styles which, despite stylistic variations, hold fast to the basic principles of the art. But there has also been a growth in the number of ways in which tai chi is practised and cross-fertilized with other systems of exercise, or spiritual pursuits (see page 31). This has led to a multiplicity of exercise systems that call themselves tai chi. As one of the classical Taoist texts from the *Tao Te Ching* says:

"The Way begets one,
One begets two,
Two begets three,
Three begets 10,000 things."

Although this short passage illustrates the amazing potential for growth and development, it may also serve as a warning to keep in mind the original idea or concept from which things originate. With so many styles – and versions of styles – in tai chi, it is becoming increasingly important that both teachers and practitioners adhere to the original principles of the art (see pages 34–5 for an explanation of the 10 basic principles of the Yang style). And, to do this, it is necessary to look back to the family styles that originated in China. If tai chi is not derived from one of the traditional family systems, it ceases to be tai chi.

Wu (Hao) style

Wu style tai chi was created by Wu Yu Xiang (1812–1880) who, like Yang Lu Chan, was a native of Yongnian County. Wu Yu Xiang and his two brothers were keen marital artists who had learned Shaolin boxing from their father. However, they were impressed by Yang Lu Chan's style of tai chi and wanted to learn it. (Wu Yu Xiang subsequently taught Yang's sons how to read and write.) Keen to develop his skills even further, Wu travelled to Chenjiagou Village to work with Yang's teacher and ended up being taught by Chen Qing Ping. His art became famous through the Hao family who learned the style from Wu's nephew, Li I Yu.

The Wu (Hao) style remains a widely recognized system of tai chi that is still taught today, both in China and in the West. It is characterized by compact, tight movements in which the practitioner can lean backward or forward (in contrast to the Yang style of tai chi in which the spine must remain vertical).

Another Wu style

Just to confuse matters, there is another Wu style of tai chi that is also widely recognized. A man called Wu Jiangquan (1870–1942) was taught by his father Wu Quan You who learned the small Yang form from Yang Lu Chan's son. This style was carried on through Wu Jiangquan's daughter Wu Ying Hwa and her husband Ma Yue Liang, who both died in the late 1990s. Their grandson Ma Jing Bao now lives in Germany and has schools in Holland, Germany and the UK.

Sun style

The most recent development in tai chi is the Sun style. This was developed in the early 1900s by Sun Lutang (1861–1930). Sun was learning Shaolin Kung-Fu and Ba Gua (an internal martial art) when he met tai chi master Hao Weichen (1849–1920) in Beijing. Sun helped Hao at a time when he was ill and needed assistance. On recovering, Hao taught Sun the Wu Yu Xiang style of tai chi. Sun went on to create his own hybrid style incorporating elements from his experiences with other martial arts.

chi – the essence of life

For thousands of years, the Chinese have believed in the existence of chi. It is the basic life force that is contained in every living thing from plants to humans. Without it we cannot exist; it is the essential energy of life and it is both inside and outside of us. Rather than having an ethereal or mystical quality, the Chinese are firmly convinced that chi is a tangible quality that is measurable.

Humans have two essential sources of chi: prenatal and postnatal. Prenatal chi is inherited from our parents and determines our basic physical health and well-being. We have no control over our prenatal chi. What we get is what we get, and some of us have a stronger constitution than others.

Postnatal chi comes from our diet and our lifestyle. By eating and drinking healthily, taking regular exercise and generally looking after ourselves we can increase our postnatal source of chi energy. Conversely, by eating unhealthy food, doing little exercise and drinking too much alcohol or smoking excessively, we deplete our postnatal chi. In the long term, this weakens the body and leads to ill health.

THE YELLOW EMPEROR

Traditional Chinese Medicine was created by the Yellow Emperor (Huang Di), who wrote the classic texts the *Nei Ching Su Wen – The Yellow Emperor's Classic of Internal Medicine*, more than 4,000 years ago. His manual was based on the theory of attaining the correct balance of yin and yang (see pages 14–16) in the body, and he mapped out the channels (meridians) in the body along which chi travels.

The river of chi

Chi travels through the body in pathways known as meridians. The meridians carry chi energy all around the body and to the main internal organs: the heart, lungs, liver, spleen and kidneys. The speed at which chi flows – and how smoothly it flows – can have a profound impact on our health and well-being.

The great benefits of tai chi (see pages 28–9) are due to the fact that its combination of movement, breathwork and mental focus both regulates and enhances the flow of chi. If your chi is blocked, sluggish or unbalanced, regular tai chi practice will bring back balance and harmony, and restore you to a state of good health.

Optimizing the flow of chi

As well as practising tai chi, there are other ways to optimize the flow of chi. Traditional Chinese Medicine incorporates a number of methods. These include: Tui Na, a Chinese massage system that uses techniques such as pressing, kneading, slapping and vibrating; Chinese herbal medicine, which uses herbs containing various qualities of yin and yang; and acupuncture, which works by inserting needles at key locations, known as acupoints (see page 26), in the body. These methods all have a positive effect on the body's flow of energy but they have one drawback in common:

RIGHT: Chi can be thought of as a river. If it flows smoothly, it nourishes the animal and plant life it contains. If it stagnates, then life within the river begins to perish. If the river flows too quickly, overflows or floods, it can destroy everything in its path.

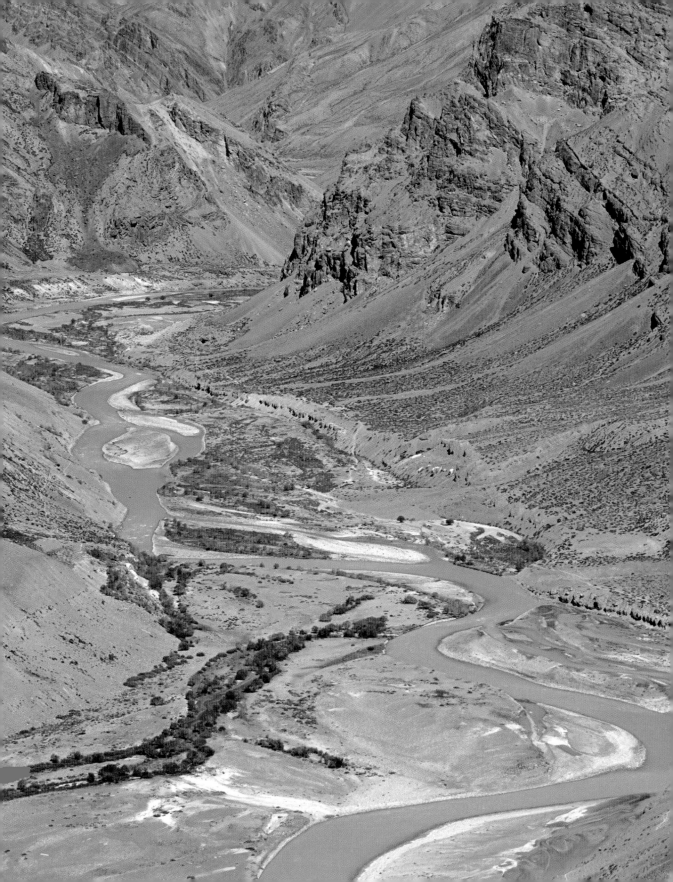

IMPORTANT ACUPOINTS

There are three acupoints on the body that are particularly important in tai chi and chi kung practice. Focusing on them during your practice can help to increase the flow of chi to these areas.

Laogong point

This point is located at the centre of the palms. Try bending your middle finger so that your fingertip rests on your palm – this is your Laogong point. Focusing here promotes the flow of chi through your hands. Students are instructed to direct their attention to this point in postures where the palms are facing, such as Turn to Catch a Ball (see page 82).

Yongquan point

This point is found on the soles of your feet (just behind the ball, in the centre). It connects to your kidney energy and is also known as the Bubbling Spring. You can concentrate on this point during standing postures to help draw up chi from the earth through the soles of your feet. The Yongquan point is also important during the sitting meditation on pages 124–5.

Beihui point

This point is located on the crown of your head. Students should focus their attention on this point at the beginning of the Form (see page 80). Imagine that you are connected to the heavens through the Beihui point. An awareness of this point ensures an upright posture and allows the spirit to rise.

they all rely on the patient putting themself in the hands of a physician. By practising tai chi, you can work on optimizing your energetic system by yourself.

Chi kung – energy work

Tai chi belongs to a huge, long-established system of exercises in China, known collectively as chi kung (also written "qigong"). "Chi" translates as "energy" and "kung" translates as "work" or "cultivation". Chi kung optimizes the flow of chi through the body in the same way as tai chi. The difference between the two is that tai chi is a martial art and chi kung is not. But many of the movements share the same slow, gentle style. Chi kung exercises are often used to warm up the body and enhance the flow of chi before a tai chi practice (many of the movements in Chapter 3 are from chi kung).

Today, it is thought that there are more than 3,000 different systems of chi kung varying in style from the simple static, standing exercises of Zhan Zhuang (see pages 70–71) to more flamboyant styles, which include Wild Goose (Dayan) chi kung and Crane chi kung. Some systems are designed as overall health-promoting exercises, while others are designed to deal with specific health problems.

A brief history of chi kung

Chi kung, of one kind or another, has been practised in China for more than 2,000 years. Although the practices are steeped in ancient culture the term "chi kung" didn't come about until the publication of a paper by Liu Gui-cheng in 1953 entitled "Practice on Qigong Therapy". Prior to this there was a diverse array of terms that were applied to energy exercises. They included Daoyin, Xingqi, Liandan, Xuangong, Jinggon, Dinggong, Xinggon, Neigong, Xiudao, Zhoshan, Neiyangong and Yangshengong.

Why practise chi kung?

Many people find that practising chi kung exercises alongside tai chi helps to awaken or enhance their sensitivity to the flow of chi.

Unlike tai chi, you don't need to learn a specific sequence of postures and transitions – you can practise chi kung postures one at a time and in no particular order. Chi kung is also an excellent way to enhance your flow of chi when you don't have enough time – or even space – to practise the tai chi Hand Form (see Chapter 4). An increased awareness of the flow of chi will inform and enrich your tai chi practice.

How tai chi and chi kung stimulate the flow of chi

There are three essential ingredients in tai chi and chi kung that help to optimize the flow of chi through the meridians in the body. These are movement, breathwork and mental focus. In combination, these three elements turn tai chi and chi kung from an exercise system into something much deeper that has benefits for the mind and spirit as well as the body.

Movement Moving the body naturally stimulates the flow of chi. If you are still, your body has no stimulus and goes into rest mode.

THE LOWER DANTIEN

Just below your navel is an area known as the lower dantien. According to Chinese tradition, this is the seat of your being – the place where chi is stored and kindled. When you breathe during tai chi or chi kung practice, you should allow your breath to descend to this area. This is the natural way that infants breathe – adults tend to take more shallow breaths that inflate the chest but not the abdomen. There are specific exercises, such as Sau Gong (see pages 72–3), that are designed to gather and store chi in your lower dantien. Sau Gong translates as "collecting the chi".

Imagine an old door that has remained closed for many years. When the door is finally opened, it needs to be gently coaxed and oiled, otherwise the hinges may snap. Likewise, if the body isn't used much, it requires consideration and care to get the chi flowing freely again. The movements of both tai chi and chi kung are specifically designed gently to increase the smooth flow of chi around the body.

If you have practised tai chi or chi kung for some time, you may experience the flow of chi as a warm or tingling sensation in a part of your body. For example, when you move your palms together in a posture, such as the chest-opening exercise on page 61, you may experience feelings of warmth or a tingling sensation in your hands. This may be quite subtle at first but, the more you practise, the more the feelings will intensify.

Breathwork Traditionally, exercise in the West has been concerned with increasing the heart rate through a fairly vigorous workout. This makes you sweat and breathe faster. In contrast, Chinese exercise systems emphasize smooth, deep, slow breathing. Students of tai chi and chi kung are taught to regulate their movements by synchronizing them with their breath. The aim is to breathe naturally and to allow your movements to match the rhythm of your breath, rather than the other way round. This helps to optimize the flow of chi.

Mental focus (yi) The third essential ingredient of chi kung and tai chi is yi, which translates as "intent" or "focus". If you do movements or exercises that you don't feel "connected to", then the overall benefits are substantially less. However, if your mind, breath and movement are all in harmony, the benefits are great. To understand the way in which your mind can affect your body, think of how you might feel in the first throes of love or when you are moved by a piece of music or a film. By applying a soft, focused intent to your tai chi or chi kung practice you will lead the chi to where it is required in your body. As the adage goes: "The mind is the governor and everything else follows."

the benefits of tai chi

Why is it that the ancient art of tai chi has survived and flourished in the 21st century? Perhaps it is because tai chi benefits not just the body, but the mind and spirit too. Among the reasons that students give for practising tai chi are greater confidence; better posture; flexibility and immunity; relief from stress and back pain; deeper and more restful sleep; and the ability to find a peaceful state of mind through meditation.

A healthy body

The health benefits of tai chi are widely backed up by both anecdotal evidence and scientific research. In Chinese medical terms, practising tai chi optimizes the flow of chi through the meridians (see page 24) and balances yin and yang energies in the body (see page 14). This, in turn, ensures that the primary internal organs – the heart, lungs, liver, spleen and kidneys – are working effectively and the immune system is strong and resilient.

When you do tai chi, you also take a little time out for yourself away from the pressure of day-to-day life. This, by itself, can help to rejuvenate your body's natural healing energy. Through being more relaxed and content, you are not constantly draining yourself with negative thoughts or emotions.

There is evidence that tai chi can help to treat a range of illnesses ranging from high blood pressure to arthritis. In addition, tai chi can play a key preventative role in healthcare. People who take up a regular tai chi practice often report suffering from fewer illnesses, such as colds and flu, than they did previously.

Better posture

A huge number of absences from work each year can be attributed to back pain which, more often than not, is the result of bad posture, lifting heavy things in the wrong way, or moving from a long period of sitting badly in a over-heated office environment to a cold outdoor environment. The regular practice of tai chi increases your awareness of your body. As you practise the postures and transitions of the tai chi Form, you will gradually discover the optimum position for sitting, standing and lifting heavy objects. These postural lessons will inform and assist you in every physical activity you do, from walking down the street to digging the garden.

Tai chi can also make you more sensitive to movements or postures that throw your body out of alignment. This awareness helps to decrease the likelihood of back injuries and pain.

Stress relief

Tai chi is renowned for its ability to help prevent and relieve stress. By paying attention to the pace of your breath, both during your practice and outside of it, you can calm extreme emotions and stay centred. The work of tai chi constantly reiterates the act of letting go on physical, psychological and emotional levels. The more you learn to loosen your body and mind, the more relaxed and peaceful you become, not just in your tai chi practice, but in the rest of your life too.

A sense of harmony

One of the main benefits to come from tai chi practice is the realization of how to achieve harmony in life. And, perhaps even more important, is the awareness you gain of the times when you start to lose harmony – this awareness allows you to take restorative action. Being in a state of harmony means that you are able to function at your best and be at peace with yourself. If you constantly push yourself too hard in your work and your personal life, eventually you will pay a price. This may come in the form of increased susceptibility to minor infections such as colds and flu, or in the form of long-term disease such as heart problems. By taking a little time each day to tune into yourself through the calm, meditative movements of tai chi you will be able to identify disharmony in your spirit.

Increased confidence

There is a direct correlation between how you use your body and how you feel emotionally. When you feel uptight, your body is tense and this is reflected in your sense of emotional well-being. If you improve your posture, you also raise your spirits and feel more confident. Just take a look at friends or colleagues who seem confident in their work and social interactions – it's unlikely that you'll find them slouching or tensing up their bodies. Confidence can stem simply from the physical act of being more

upright and relaxed. Try copying the postures on the left – observe the effect that each one has on your mood.

A healthy old age

In the future, there will be a greater number of older people than ever before. This has created concerns about how an ageing population in declining health can be supported and cared for. Continuing to have a strong, healthy body in old age will be increasingly important for everyone. Tai chi is a system of exercise that offers health benefits to people of all ages for the whole of their life. Owing to the nature of the slow, controlled movements, you can practise tai chi up until the end of your life. Many tai chi practitioners have maintained a healthy body and a sharp mind until their later years, often until their middle to late 90s. Even if you have never practised tai chi before, there is no reason why you cannot start in later life. You don't have to be in peak physical fitness and you can progress gently at the right pace for you.

Scientific studies in the West have found that tai chi has the following benefits for health in older people: it helps to reduce blood pressure and the incidence of accidental falls; it improves balance and aerobic capacity; and it helps people who have had a stroke to recover damaged functions.

Spiritual development

Tai chi can be a path to spiritual growth. It has often been described as a moving meditation and you may find it easier to reach a meditative state through tai chi than through other forms of meditation that require you to sit still. Once you are familiar with the movements of tai chi you will find that you are able to stop thinking about what you are doing and reach a place beyond thought – and eventually beyond space and time – in which you experience a sense of oneness.

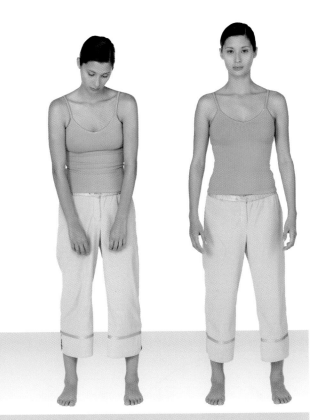

LEFT: Tai chi teaches you how an open, relaxed posture can affect your mood and sense of well-being. Standing in a closed, tense posture (see far left) has a negative effect on your mood and self-confidence. Whereas letting your body relax and open out (see near left) immediately improves the way you feel.

tai chi today

Tai chi has become incredibly popular in the last 30 to 40 years and many different styles have emerged. Because of this proliferation in styles, there are now tai chi courses to suit people across the board, from serious martial artists at one end to older people recovering from heart problems at the other.

Tai chi for health

Although all systems of tai chi have strong health benefits, many of the traditional systems are physically demanding and require long periods of sustained practice. Many contemporary students are looking for a more simple exercise routine in which they can get health benefits from a fairly short practice two or three times a week. The form of tai chi created by Cheng Man Ching (see box) is a modification of the original Yang style and it takes approximately 10 minutes to complete (rather than the 25 minutes required for the Yang Long Form). This routine, and others like it, have enjoyed an upsurge in interest as the need for shorter, simpler approaches to tai chi has grown. Most of the courses offered by health centres, colleges, and health promotion departments teach these shortened forms. (The style in Chapter 4 of this book is the first section of the Cheng Man Ching Form.)

THE CHENG MAN CHING SHORT YANG FORM

This style of tai chi is very popular in the West (some of the postures are featured in Chapter 4). Cheng Man Ching (1900–1975) took up the art on the advice of his uncle after contracting tuberculosis in his early 30s. He became a student of Yang Chen Fu in Shanghai, and was renowned as a Master of Five Excellences: painting, poetry, calligraphy, medicine and tai chi.

Cheng Man Ching did much to promote tai chi in Taiwan where he taught the wife of Chiang Kai-shek (the Chinese Nationalist leader; 1887–1975). Having seen the effectiveness of the art, Chen Kai Chek instructed Cheng Man Ching to teach his army the martial applications of tai chi. As he was given little time to train the soldiers in the Long Yang Form – which consisted of 108 movements – Cheng shortened the sequence to a 37-step Short Form. This change went on to make tai chi accessible to many who previously did not have time to learn the traditional system.

In the mid-1960s, Cheng moved to the US and began teaching his shortened routine to Westerners. This was the first time that the art had been openly taught in the West and the new Short Form was well suited to Westerners who had less time (and perhaps less patience) to devote to tai chi. After teaching in San Francisco, Cheng moved to New York where he established a school, teaching what has become an internationally famous lineage of tai chi. His students come from all over the world.

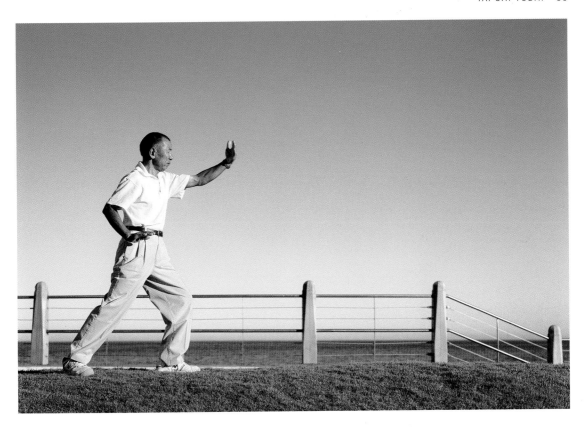

People's Republic Forms

In 1956, the Chinese government created a modified set of postures from the Yang style of tai chi (see pages 21–2). They dispensed with the more difficult postures and cut out some repetitions, making the original 108-movement Long Form into a more manageable 24 postures.

Competition routines

In 1979, the Chinese State Physical Education and Sports Commission created a competition routine, which included the strongest characteristics from the traditional Chen, Yang and Wu family styles of tai chi (see pages 20–23), as well as aspects of the more flamboyant Wushu routines. This gave rise to the now popular 48-movement tai chi Form.

Some traditionalists lament the watering down of the original styles of tai chi but, in competition terms, the advantages are that shortened forms can be more dynamic, they help to hold the attention of judges and they may also be more visually appealing to spectators.

ABOVE: Many people learn tai chi not because they want to be dedicated martial artists, but because they seek a peaceful mind and a balanced body. The demand for short forms of tai chi that can be integrated into a busy lifestyle has grown dramatically.

Tailor-made tai chi

Some tai chi routines have been created with a specific aim in mind. One example of this is a programme developed by Dr Paul Lam, a Chinese man resident in Australia. Dr Lam's program is specifically geared to help people with arthritis. He teaches people an eight-step Form over a few weekends. It is likely that other truncated systems will appear as tai chi is adapted for more groups of people with specific needs.

Some classes taught in gyms and health clubs "borrow" tai chi movements and sequences and integrate them with other forms of exercise to create a kind of tai chi hybrid. Examples of this are Chi Ball and Body Balance classes, which teach a combination of tai chi, yoga and Pilates. These bear little relation to the tai chi that you would be taught in a dedicated tai chi class.

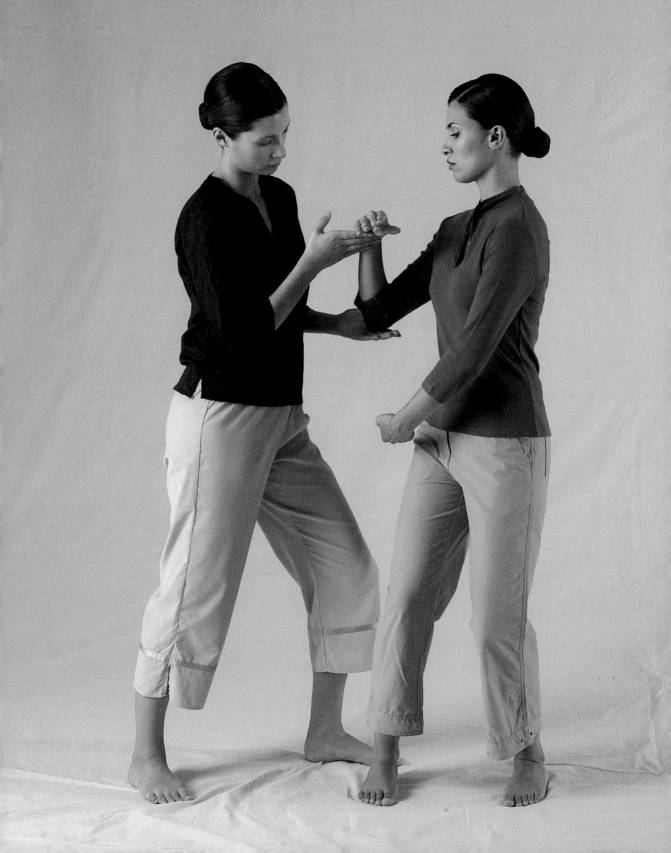

how to practise

Tai chi isn't just about moving through a series of postures – it's about creating harmony between your mind, your breath and your body. As you become familiar with the movements of tai chi, you will start to have a greater awareness of your physical and emotional state. You'll be able to observe disharmony quickly and take steps to correct it.

In this chapter I explain some of the techniques that inform the practice of tai chi, such as correct posture, groundedness and letting go of tension. An understanding of these things will help you to tune in to your body and get a deeper sense of its workings. It will also guide and enrich your tai chi practice. Toward the end of the chapter, I provide some practical guidelines for beginning tai chi, whether you choose to go to classes or practise by yourself at home.

ten principles of tai chi

Although there are many different styles of tai chi, you can apply these 10 principles from the Yang style of tai chi (see pages 21–2) to most styles – they are the basic tools of the art. Take some time to understand what each one means and, with patience, apply it to your practice. Rather than learning all 10 at once, it is a good idea to read and think about each principle one at a time. Each time you practise tai chi, introduce a new principle and make it the focus of your routine. Eventually, you will be able to integrate all 10 into your practice.

1. Lift your head and raise your spirit

When you practise tai chi, hold your head up straight without tension. Keep your neck relaxed to allow blood and chi to circulate freely. You can keep your head in this position by imagining an object balanced on top of it. Try also to be aware of other parts of your head, such as your face, mouth and eyes. Keep your face relaxed, and inhale through your nose and exhale through your mouth. Gently touch your tongue to the roof of your mouth as you inhale. Let your eyes follow the movements of your hands. Visualize yourself suspended from a string like a puppet. Cultivate a sense of yourself as youthful, alive and full of vitality and spirit.

2. Settle your shoulders and drop your elbows

Let your shoulders relax and settle into their natural position. If you allow your shoulders to relax, your elbows should naturally drop down and point to the ground. This gives you power and facilitates a good flow of chi. If you don't relax, you will become tense and waste energy and power. Don't direct power from your upper body in an upward direction; instead use internal strength originating from your centre (the lower dantien; see page 27) below your navel.

3. Relax your chest and pluck your back

Rather than pushing your chest out, let it relax and sink inward slightly – this reduces the pressure on your lungs and naturally facilitates deep, relaxed breathing. This gentle movement also helps to stimulate the surrounding organs in a healthy way. When your chest is relaxed and sunk slightly, your back will naturally assume the correct raised position (tai chi practitioners refer to this as "plucking the back"). This allows energy to settle in the lower dantien and increases your effectiveness during pushing movements (for example, see page 89).

4. Loosen your waist and relax your hips

Loosening and relaxing your waist and hips are essential in tai chi. This is because of all your movement should begin from your waist. By relaxing your waist, you will naturally have greater stability, a strong foundation and good control of your legs during the shift from empty to full, or insubstantial to substantial (see following principle). Avoid unnatural or forced waist movements – they will make you lose power, control and accuracy.

5. Apply the principle of "substantial" and "insubstantial"

The terms "substantial" and "insubstantial" refer to the weight that you carry in your legs. During your practice you are continually shifting your weight so that when one leg "empties" of weight or becomes insubstantial, the other one becomes "full" of weight or substantial. The insubstantial leg can easily change direction because all the weight is in the other leg. To explore this, try the stepping exercise on pages 78–9.

6. Harmonize your upper and lower body movements

Harmony of movement is an important aspect of tai chi. An old tai chi adage states: "The root is in the feet, dispensed through the legs, controlled by the waist, and orchestrated in the fingers." When energy moves from your feet, up your legs and to your waist, your gaze should follow the movements – this will help your entire body to move in harmony. If one part of your body stops completely and another continues, the harmony is broken and instead there is chaos.

7. Use the mind, not force

Among tai chi practitioners it is often said: "Lead entirely with your mind, do not use force in movement." When practising tai chi, there should be nothing rigid or forceful about your body or your movements. Your entire body should be relaxed rather than stiff. This includes your joints and veins, as well as your muscles. For example, your hands should be so relaxed that none of your veins and tendons stand out (this is referred to as "beautiful lady's hands"). Any stiffness will inhibit the flow of energy.

To lead with your mind means that wherever your attention goes, energy will follow. To apply this in tai chi, you need to focus your attention on and visualize the movement that you are about to make. The following technique, used in Zen archery, illustrates the principle of leading with your mind.

In Zen archery the archer doesn't aim for the target; instead his body lines up with the target and he aligns his mind to the path of the arrow. In a sense, the archer creates the arrow's path by putting his mind there and allowing the arrow to follow. When you are performing tai chi, although your mind is still, it remains focused on what you are doing. This mental focus allows your tai chi practice to develop quickly – and the benefits of relaxation and focus will spill over into your daily life. Whether you are studying for an exam or working on an important business project there comes a point where you have done all the training, and you know what needs to be done. If you visualize your "target" and allow your mind to lead, you can achieve a great deal.

8. Harmonize the internal and the external

In tai chi your mind and spirit lead and your body is the follower. If your mind and spirit are tranquil, your body will be light, graceful and alive. To bring harmony between the physical and the internal is to achieve completeness in tai chi.

If you find yourself practising tai chi while thinking about your job, or something that is causing you stress, it's far better to take the time to clear your mind and then come back to your training later. Imagine trying to score a goal in football when worrying about a work deadline. Despite the fact that your body might be fit and capable of scoring the goal, the chances are that you would miss. Whatever you are doing, you will be more successful if you are in a peaceful state of mind. Giving half your mind to something is ultimately counterproductive.

9. Understand continuity

In many hard-style martial arts, such as karate, a movement has a beginning and an end. It is in the space between the end of one movement and the beginning of another, that the student is vulnerable to attack. This is because stopping and starting interrupts the flow of energy around the body. Tai chi differs from other martial arts in that a movement does not stop, it just changes direction. The flowing movements of tai chi can be compared to a great river or to silk unravelling from a cocoon.

10. Seek serenity in motion

Hard-style or "external" martial arts often involve high-energy moves, such as jumping or spinning. The disadvantage of these actions is that they can take you out of your centre. This leaves you open and vulnerable to your opponent. In tai chi, you work to remain calm and serene throughout your practice. In training with a calm, relaxed mind you are in a better position to rationally respond to any kind of attack, whether physical, mental or emotional. Your breathing is deeper and more controlled, and you can concentrate on sinking energy to the lower dantien (see page 27). Your mind, body and pulse all remain calm.

letting go of tension

One of the primary reasons people come to tai chi classes is because they want to get rid of tension. Tai chi can certainly help to alleviate tension but, ironically, it would be so much better if students came to the class relaxed in the first place. Approaching the art of tai chi in a relaxed, open way makes the learning process much easier.

The right amount of tension

A certain amount of tension is essential to allow you to move and function efficiently. For example, if your body was 100 per cent relaxed, you wouldn't be able to stand up. Yet, if there is too much tension located in any part of your body, you move less effectively and you may start to experience discomfort and pain. Finding the right balance is important in tai chi. The following exercise will help you to discover how little tension you need in your body.

Take a few minutes to stand still. Stand with your feet shoulder-distance apart and your toes pointing slightly inward so that the outsides of your feet are parallel. Soften your knees. Now close your eyes. Allow yourself to listen to your breath. Don't try to change it – just feel where it is in your body and how it affects your body. Allow your breath to soften slowly and find its way to settling in your lower abdomen.

Now think about how you are standing. Consider the miracle of one bone resting on another in order to create the erect, upright human frame. Don't strive for total stillness – be aware of the little dance that goes on inside your body as it tries to find the best way to support itself. Be aware of when you start to grip or hold onto yourself in order to maintain stability. Think about how the weight of your body doesn't merely rest on the surface of the floor but sinks downward, through the ground, into the heart of the earth. Imagine relaxing your body from the inside, rather than externally.

A good way to relax from the inside is to visualize the inside of your body as an egg-timer in which the minute grains of sand are slowly trickling through the tiny hole in the middle. Imagine the grains of sand settling in the lower half of your body and then sinking down toward the earth. Meanwhile, your upper body becomes light and open. You can also visualize your upper body floating freely like a balloon. If you practise using these images, you will discover how your body can support itself while also relaxing on a very deep level.

Swinging your arms

This is another simple exercise that gives you a sense of where and how you hold tension in your body. Stand up, find your equilibrium and let your arms hang by your sides. Now, slowly turn at your waist from one side to the other. Observe what happens to your arms – the more relaxed you are, the more freely your arms will move with your body. If your body is free from tension, your arms will follow the momentum of your waist a bit like the way the ribbons of a maypole turn with the pole.

Learning to let go

Once you are aware of tension and the impact it can have upon your body – and your emotions (see page 29) – you can begin the work of overcoming it. The concept of "letting go" is an important part of tai chi. Through the work of tai chi you can start to let go of anything that is unnecessary or increases your burden in life. This can range from overcoming bad postural habits to letting go of resentment in a personal relationship.

RIGHT: Getting rid of physical and emotional tension is integral to tai chi. Imagining that you are connected to the sky and the heavens through your upper body can free you.

the importance of posture

One of the major benefits of tai chi is the positive impact it has on your posture. Through the course of their working lives, many people develop poor postural habits. When your posture is poor, everything that has to travel through your body – oxygen, nutrients and chi – needs to work much harder to do its job. When your posture is good, your body will be healthy, relaxed and open, and it will work better. You will look and feel good too.

The work of tai chi inspires you to consider, on a very deep level, the structure of your body. By improving your awareness of posture, you can begin to understand how best your body can support itself in a relaxed and effective manner.

Many high-level tai chi instructors emphasize that the most important posture a student can learn is simply standing still (the "attention" position). The following exercise is a more detailed version of the exercise on page 36. Stand with your feet shoulder-distance apart and your toes pointing slightly inward so that the outsides of your feet are parallel. Soften your knees. Now close your eyes and pay attention to the following.

• Your breath: listen to the breath flowing in and out of your body and try to become aware of any tightness or impediments in the flow of air. Allow your breathing to become smooth and settle in your lower abdomen. Take time to let this happen naturally. Focus your attention inward.

• Small movements: feel your body move slightly from side to side or forward and backward as your body finds the best way to position itself in an upright position. Allow these movements to occur and quietly follow where they take you. Eventually, your body will find the best position to allow you to be motionless.

• Aches and pains: it is normal to get small aches and pains from time to time. They are nature's way of telling you that you need to pay attention to a particular part of your body. Mentally scan your body for little areas of discomfort, and try to sense what adjustments you need to make to alleviate them and facilitate

good posture. Areas of discomfort often result from a misalignment of the body that has developed over many years – for example, constantly carrying a heavy bag on the same shoulder can distort your posture and cause pain.

• Noise: be aware of all the little distractions that are going on around you, such as the distant noise of traffic, machinery or people's voices. We all grimace when hearing extremely loud sounds such as a road being drilled, yet smaller, less intrusive sounds can also take their toll on us in a more insidious way. Start by being aware of your body's reaction to sounds in your environment. Feel how they take you away from yourself. Over time, "let go" of the noises around you by bringing your attention inward and allowing yourself to relax.

Ergonomic effectiveness

The body can be used efficiently or inefficiently. An important principle in tai chi is to do as little as possible and let things go their own natural way. This doesn't mean lying around doing nothing – it means cultivating a sense of how little is required for your body to do its work effectively.

Imagine you have just been given the job of sweeping a main street. Not, perhaps the most pleasant of tasks I know, but bear with me. It's your first day on the job and you've been told you have three hours to clean a three-mile stretch before lunch. After this you must move on to another location. You may start off feeling fairly relaxed – the weather is fine and there's not too much

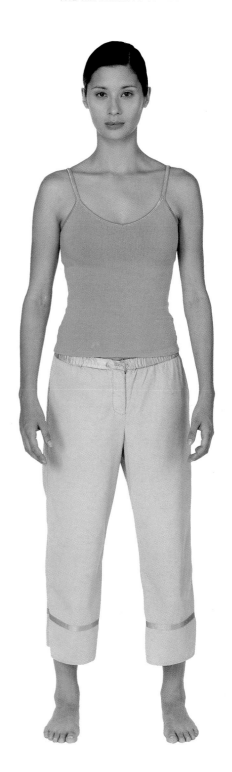

rubbish around. An hour later, you're less than half-way through the job and the litter seems to be increasing with every step. Soon you become frantic and move predominantly from your shoulders and upper body, as you sweep in short, sharp movements. Compare this to the man who has done the job for 30 years. Over the years he has cultivated a relaxed and mindful way of working. He knows very clearly what is required of him and how long the job will take. In fact, he doesn't even think about the work – his body has found its own natural way of moving the brush and he can complete the task with little or no physical tension. The more we train to do something, the better we become at it. It is as simple as that.

In tai chi, you learn to move from the central position of your body – through your waist – and the rest of your body follows naturally. There is no superfluous movement – you never move your arms in isolation while keeping your body still. Your whole body moves as one with a direct correlation between your upper and lower torso. Through regular tai chi practice, you will learn ergonomic effectiveness. Soon this will impact on your life outside of your tai chi sessions. You'll find that you can apply your awareness of good posture to a range of situations and activities from standing still to mowing the lawn to lifting heavy objects.

RIGHT: The attention posture is widely considered the most important in tai chi. This is where you turn your attention inward and let go of discomfort, tension and distraction.

grounding

The concept of grounding in tai chi is very important. Keeping your weight and energy centred in your lower body and letting your upper body become light and free allows you to move with sensitivity and accuracy. Being grounded not only helps during your tai chi practice, but in the rest of life too. If you are grounded, you can deal with life's problems calmly and with equanimity.

Being grounded

We all know what it is like to feel ungrounded. It's a sensation that has both a physical and an emotional reality – and one feeds into the other. Imagine that you've taken on a big mortgage and your boss tells you that you are being made redundant. It is likely that your breath would quicken and your heart would pump fast. Your energy would surge to the upper part of your body and you would start to feel out of control.

Being grounded means, quite literally, being connected to the ground or the earth. It means keeping your energy centred in your lower body and feeling rooted to the ground through your feet. Imagine a plant – its roots are firmly embedded in the earth where they gather sustenance, while the upper part of the plant is light and able to move in the wind. The roots of the plant are yang and the upper part of the plant is yin (see pages 14–16).

Ideally, we should have the same distribution of yin and yang as a plant. Our upper body should be yin and our lower body should be yang. But life in today's Western technological society means that, for many of us, the polarity of nature is reversed: our upper bodies and minds have become increasingly yang and our lower bodies increasingly yin. This has happened because, today, most people make their living using minimal physical exertion. Our minds are constantly active and our bodies are virtually inactive (with the exception of the upper-body movements involved in driving or using a keyboard). In the past this was different: human work usually consisted of physical labour that helped to keep the body active and the mind free from stress.

The grounding effect of tai chi

Apart from the emotional consequences of being ungrounded, there are physical side-effects too. Because of an emphasis on repetitive upper-body movements, many people tend to suffer from an accumulation of tension in the upper body which results in backache, shoulder pain, and headache.

Tai chi teaches you to empty your mind, free your upper body, keep your energy settled in your lower body and to feel rooted to the ground. Emotionally, this makes you feel stable and calm. Physically, it helps you to move in the most efficient way and prevents tension and discomfort in your upper body.

Staying grounded in everyday life

When you become experienced at tai chi you can apply its principles in your everyday life. Imagine, for example, that you are encountering verbal abuse. If you try to out-talk or out-shout your opponent, you rob yourself of the sensitivity that could help you find solutions. An alternative approach is to respond to aggression by remaining quiet, calm and grounded. This enables you to hear the other person's point of view and deal with the problem in a clear, rational way. It also allows the other person's anger to dissipate. The practice of tai chi provides a basis from which to develop this kind of grounded response.

RIGHT: Visualizing solid, stable objects from nature, such as rocks, tree roots or mountains, can help you to cultivate a sense of rootedness and groundedness.

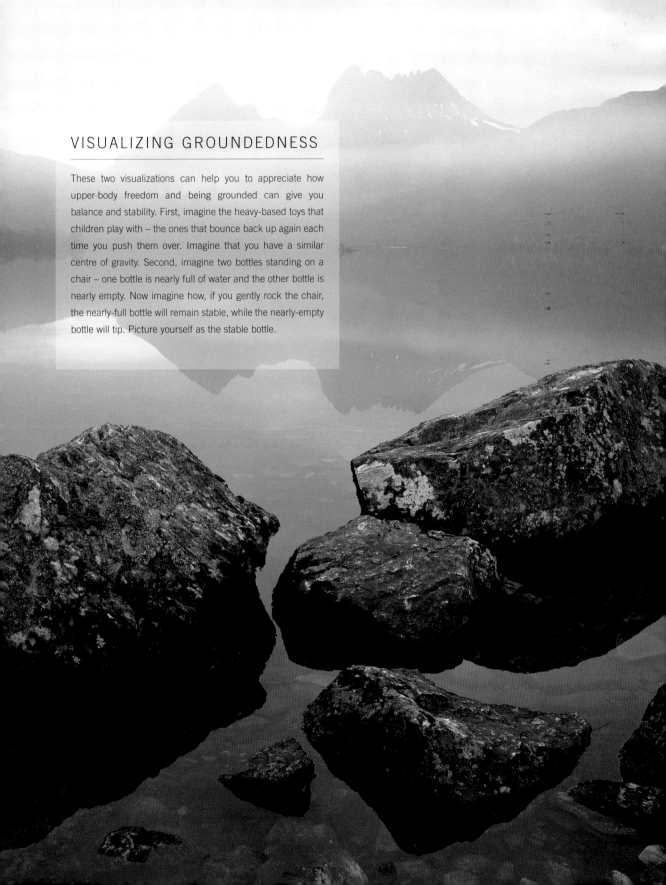

VISUALIZING GROUNDEDNESS

These two visualizations can help you to appreciate how upper-body freedom and being grounded can give you balance and stability. First, imagine the heavy-based toys that children play with – the ones that bounce back up again each time you push them over. Imagine that you have a similar centre of gravity. Second, imagine two bottles standing on a chair – one bottle is nearly full of water and the other bottle is nearly empty. Now imagine how, if you gently rock the chair, the nearly-full bottle will remain stable, while the nearly-empty bottle will tip. Picture yourself as the stable bottle.

ting jing

Ting Jing is a term that means "listening energy". It is the art of listening, not just with your ears, but with all of your bodily senses. Developing an increased awareness of yourself, others and your environment is one of the most powerful things you can gain from tai chi.

Learning to listen with your body is not a skill that can be reduced to a set of tips or techniques. When you first start to practise tai chi, listening energy may not be a concept that seems particularly meaningful or relevant to you. Yet, as you continue your practice, you may notice that your senses and your awareness of your surroundings naturally become more acute. The following two legendary tales are good illustrations of the principle of Ting Jing. The greater your understanding of listening energy, the better you can recognize and cultivate it in yourself.

Ting Jing and physical relaxation

A tai chi master was practising in the park one morning. His mind was calm and relaxed and the air was still. He had blended so well into his environment that a bird landed on his shoulder. When the bird tried to fly off it couldn't. No matter how hard it tried, it was unable to take flight. The master had developed his listening skill to such a level that he could discern exactly how much pressure the bird was applying in order to push off to take flight. By knowing this, the master was able to relax his body just enough to absorb the pressure of the poor, bewildered bird.

Ting Jing and avoiding attack

Another tai chi master was renowned throughout his province for his martial prowess. For 40 years, he was the undefeated champion in his region. A young man was so keen to beat the old master that he practised regularly for eight hours a day for six months. One evening, the young man was returning home from his training session and saw the old master working in the fields. As he stooped down low over his seedlings he seemed like an easy target. The young student slowly crept up behind him and, when he felt he was close enough, took the opportunity to pounce on the old man. At that precise moment, the old master turned round and threw the young man across the field. The angry young man couldn't believe what had happened. "How is that possible?" he exclaimed. "I have diligently trained every day for eight hours, for the past six months and yet you defeated my surprise attack with great ease. How much time do you spend training?"

"Every waking moment," replied the old master. Because the master had allowed his training to become his life, his listening ability had been honed to the point at which he knew how little or how much movement was needed – and when – in order that he might avoid attack.

Cultivating Ting Jing

To cultivate listening energy, get into the habit of tuning in to yourself whenever you have the opportunity. Start off by being still and quiet – closing your eyes if you can – and bringing your awareness to your breath. Once you have a sense of your breath, stay connected to it. Focus your awareness on your lower abdomen. Then turn your attention to what is around you. Feel the temperature of your environment; feel the breeze if you are outside; and listen to the sounds in your environment. Many of us are constantly surrounded by sounds, colours and movement. Notice how different aspects of your environment affect you – some may please you, while others may disturb you. By taking this time to tune in to yourself, you will begin to develop skills that will serve you well in the art of Ting Jing.

Ultimately, listening energy must be practised with another person. Ting Jing is the sense of listening to the qualities of others and intuiting how they relate to you. It begins with physical contact but ultimately transcends the physical. To understand this better, think back to a time when you have walked into a room of people and sensed an energy or atmosphere – either positive or negative. It is this kind of sensitivity in all your interactions with others that you are working toward cultivating in tai chi.

To cultivate listening energy with a partner, try the Sticking Hands exercises on pages 112–13. In Tui Shou (Pushing Hands; see pages 114–15), be attentive to your partner's movement and energy. Instead of relying on sight to gauge your partner's intention, use your listening ability (try closing your eyes and see how this affects your responses). Try to sense how much weight they are moving toward you. This enables you to respond with exactly the right amount of movement. When you are working with a partner try to let go of any feelings of aggression or competition that you might be harbouring. To develop listening energy you both need be in a peaceful state of mind. If you and your partner work together with a sense of mutual support, cooperation and exploration, you will speed up the learning process.

BELOW: When you have cultivated Ting Jing you will be able to stand in nature and be perfectly attuned and at one with your environment.

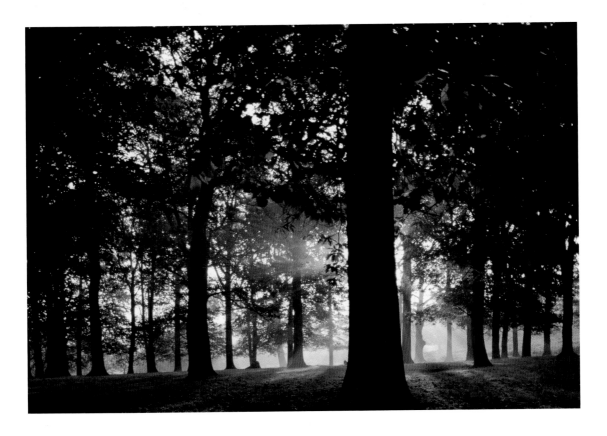

tai chi classes

Many people who practise tai chi enjoy the discipline, structure and social aspects of attending classes. If you are just beginning tai chi, the advantages of going to a class are that your teacher will set the pace for your learning, give you precise information about the position of your hands and feet, and correct any mistakes you make. It can also be helpful and inspiring to see the postures performed by someone who has been practising tai chi for many years.

How to find a class

There are many approaches to and interpretations of tai chi – even if a class contains elements of tai chi, it doesn't necessarily teach a traditional range of postures. For example, some classes teach a hybrid of tai chi, yoga and Pilates (see page 31). To find an authentic tai chi class, it is a good idea to seek information from a recognized authority (see page 138). You will find that there are many registered instructors teaching a range of classes in a variety of locations. When choosing a class, you need to know what your primary motivation is for learning tai chi – some classes are focused on improving health and relieving stress. Other classes treat tai chi as a martial art and include partner-work and/or weapons training.

How often to attend

You should aim to attend a class for at least one or two hours per week. Obviously, if you are able to attend classes more frequently than this, you will learn faster and feel the benefits more quickly. However, a class is where you learn the mechanics of the movements and postures – ultimately, it is the practice that you do by yourself at home that will lead to the deepest understanding of tai chi.

If you have difficulty attending classes, some teachers offer private tuition. Working one-to-one with a qualified teacher allows you to learn quickly, but there is more onus on you to practise regularly. You can't hide at the back of the class if you haven't trained on a particular week!

The venue

As well as martial art schools, tai chi classes are now held in offices, universities, health clubs and lots of other community spaces. Choose a location that feels right for you – somewhere that is easy to get to on a regular basis and somewhere that feels comfortable and peaceful. Ideally, you should practise away from noise, and other distractions, and in a place where there is a flow of clean, fresh air.

What to expect from a class

It's common to start a class with some loosening exercises. These will both open and relax your body while promoting the flow of chi (energy) through your meridians. They may be general warm-up exercises or they may be chi kung exercises (see Chapter 3 for some examples). Your teacher may also guide you through some exercises designed to increase your body awareness and sensitivity. For example, you may be encouraged to bring your attention to various points in your body while visualizing your connection to the heavens through your mind and the ground through your feet.

Next, your tai chi teacher will teach the postures of the Hand Form (see Chapter 4). You will be given guidance about the exact position of your arms, hands, feet and body. If you are in a beginners' class, you should be taught the postures a few at a time. As the postures become familiar to you, you will be encouraged to perform them as a fluid sequence with no obvious beginning and end to each posture.

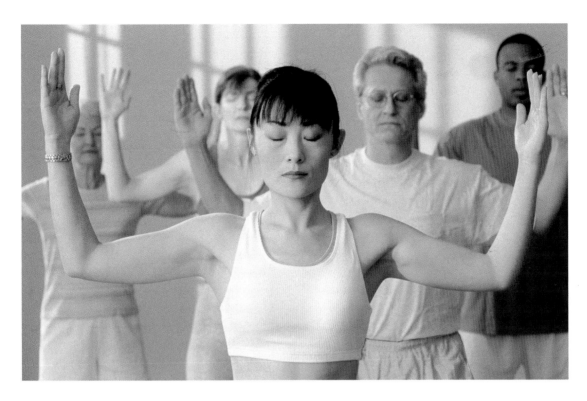

ABOVE: It's important to focus inward during a tai chi class. The lessons of tai chi come from listening to the information that comes to you internally each time you move through a posture.

The question of etiquette varies from teacher to teacher. Classes tend to be informal, open and friendly with little ritual or ceremony. In some classes, teachers may bow to students before and after each session and the bow is returned by the students. This is more a mark of mutual respect than a strict discipline.

Putting aside ego

Often, in mixed-level classes, students start with good intentions and study the early postures well. However, problems can begin when the ego kicks in and they want to be at a level that is beyond their ability. I recommend that you clearly understand each sequence before progressing to the next. This means being able to perform the movements without having to think about them. Once you are familiar with the geography of each posture you can focus on what you are doing, rather than how you are doing it.

SHORT TAI CHI COURSES

A short tai chi course (usually 8 to 10 weeks) can provide an excellent introduction to the art. But it's important to realize that the benefits gained from a short course are very different from those of joining an ongoing tai chi class in which students are trained over a period of years. Short courses often concentrate on teaching only the Hand Form of tai chi, which is only one side of this multi-faceted art. As you will discover later in this book, there are many associated exercises that can inform your practice of the Hand Form and help to give you a deeper understanding of tai chi. Ideally, you should learn tai chi over a long period of time so that you can assimilate information slowly and gently.

tai chi at home

It's easy to practise tai chi at home – you don't need any special tools or equipment – you just need some space, and the motivation to practise on a regular basis. One of the great advantages of doing tai chi at home is that you have the opportunity to fully tune in to your mind, body and spirit, without any distractions.

Creating a daily practice

You will benefit most from tai chi if you practise on a daily basis – preferably for the same duration at the same time every day. Think carefully about when you can train and for how long – you need to be able to fit your practice into your usual routine. If you set yourself unrealistic goals, you'll find it difficult to maintain your tai chi practice in the long term. Even practising for as little as 10 minutes a day is fine at first. Aim to let the art become as regular a part of your life as eating, drinking and sleeping.

You will be most inspired to practise tai chi if you create a peaceful, relaxed environment that you can enjoy being in. If your home is distractingly noisy, it can help to play some soft, unobtrusive music. If your lighting is harsh, try practising in natural light or light some candles. You do not need a large room in which to practise tai chi. Even if you are in a very small space and find that your movement is restricted, you can modify the size of the steps you take when you practise the Hand Form (see Chapter 4).

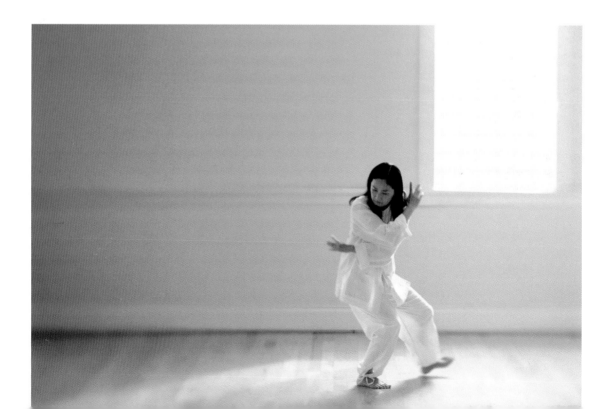

Clothing

Try to avoid tight, restrictive clothing, particularly around your waist. If you wear soft fabrics, you will get a clearer sense of how each transition affects the movement of your clothes. You should also wear thin-soled flat shoes or work barefoot so you can feel each gradual transference from one foot to the other.

Visualize the postures

When you teach yourself tai chi at home, you will need to look carefully at the photographs in Chapter 4 and get a clear idea of the position your feet should be in (the grids beneath each photograph will help you to do this). You should also observe the position of the arms in relation to the model's body and how the shoulders are always relaxed and down (even when the model's arms are raised).

Before you try the positions of the Hand Form in Chapter 4, try to be really clear in your mind's eye what they look like. By holding a clear mental image of each posture in your mind, they will be easier to replicate. The worst thing you can do is to get a rough idea of the postures and try to move forward more than your ability really allows.

When you get into a posture, try to find the best stance for your individual height and body shape by moving your weight slightly forward, backward and side to side. Come to rest in the position that feels right for you.

Warm up first

It can be tempting to go straight into a tai chi practice without warming up first, especially if you are short of time. Warm-up exercises are as important for the mind as they are for the body. For example, if you go from a busy day straight into doing tai chi,

OPPOSITE: Practising tai chi by yourself at home brings long-lasting benefits. Try to make your practice sessions enjoyable rather than a chore. This way you won't be tempted to give up when life gets busy or stressful.

your attention is likely to be scattered and your mind buzzing. You won't experience the full benefits of the practice while in this state. If, on the other hand, you begin with some of the chi kung exercises in Chapter 3, you are more likely to practise the Hand Form in a mindful, meditative way.

Overcoming problems

When you practise tai chi by yourself it is up to you rather than a teacher to set the pace at which you work. If you find that you are moving through the postures in Chapter 4 very quickly, make an effort to slow down. The slower you do tai chi, the better. If you slow down your breathing, this will help you to move your arms and legs at a slower pace. Chi kung exercises are good for encouraging slow, deep breathing.

Staying motivated

If you remind yourself of the potential benefits that can be gained from regular practice, then you will be more determined to train. Try to create a space just for you and your practice and ask your family and friends to help you to honour this precious time. Don't eat a large meal beforehand, but don't let yourself be hungry either. Disconnect your telephone and let some natural air into your space. Take the time to acclimatize to your surroundings and connect to your breath before you begin.

If you have mobility problems, don't push yourself too far. Work within your limits and in time you will be able to gently extend your range of movement. Try to pay close attention to the physical sensations of your body and remember that pain is nature's way of telling you that something is not right. If you feel discomfort – perhaps sore knees or slight pain in the lower back – pay closer attention to how you are standing and moving from one foot to the other.

Before and after each training session, spend a few minutes tuning in to how you feel. This will give you a clear sense of how your training is progressing. Remember one thing – above all tai chi should be enjoyable!

beginning the hand form

When people think of tai chi, they usually think of someone performing a sequence of slow, graceful movements that flow seamlessly into one other. This is the Form, or the Hand Form. Although it's possible also to practise tai chi with a partner or using weapons, the basic Hand Form, performed alone, is where your training is likely to start. Your challenge is to become as familiar as you can with the movements and transitions of the Hand Form – to learn them so well that you can do them without thinking.

The exact number and type of postures in the tai chi Hand Form differs depending on what style of tai chi you choose to do (see pages 20–23). Even within one style of tai chi, there are short and long versions of the Hand Form. For example, in the Yang style of tai chi, the Long Yang Form consists of 108 steps, whereas a modified version – the Short Yang Form – consists of 37 steps. The postures that follow in Chapter 4 (starting on page 80) are from the opening section of the Short Yang Form, as devised by Cheng Man Ching (see page 30). They will provide you with a taste of what tai chi can offer.

One step at a time

When students are presented with a fairly short sequence of postures, they often have a tendency to try to memorize it in its entirety and do it all at once. A far better approach is to study one or two postures and practise them over and over again. When you can perform these smoothly, and without asking yourself "what comes next?", build the next one or two postures into the sequence in the same way. Continue like this until you have mastered all of the postures.

The following analogy illustrates the degree of familiarity that I recommend you establish in the process of learning tai chi. Imagine that you've just returned from your favourite flat-pack furniture store with a beautiful new wardrobe. Picture yourself trying to assemble it by either ignoring the instructions, or just paying them a cursory glance. It is more than likely that you'll have a frustrating few hours ahead of you and a pretty shaky piece of furniture. Now, instead, imagine that you sit down and study the instructions. Each step of the process is clear in your head before you attempt it. Rather than being in a rush to do everything at once, you apply your complete concentration to each stage of construction. The chances are that putting the wardrobe together in this way will be much less stressful, and the end result will be more solid and durable.

On average it takes students a year to learn a Hand Form (less with committed and intensive training), and a Hand Form takes between 3 and 20 minutes to perform. When you have learned the postures in Chapter 4, they should take you around 3 minutes. By repeating the postures in Chapter 4 four or five times in one session, you will get many of the same benefits that you would from practising a longer version of the Hand Form.

Repetition is the key

It is not merely executing the postures of the Hand Form with skill and accuracy that provides the benefits of tai chi; it is also the constant repetition of postures. Repetition gradually re-educates our bodies and minds and helps us develop a whole new way of moving and being. As you increase your familiarity with the postures, all of your previous postural and behavioural habits will change for the better.

An awareness of yin and yang

Rather than concentrating solely on the physical position of your body, let an awareness of yin and yang inform the way you practise. Remind yourself of the respective qualities of yin and yang (see pages 14–16) and apply them to each posture – try to work toward a balance of hardness and softness, movement and stillness, and strength and yielding. Tai chi can encompass these apparent contradictions. For example, as you move your waist, arms and legs, you will begin to have a sense of your mind and your internal organs remaining still. Tai chi is often referred to as "stillness in motion".

As your awareness of yin and yang develops, you will discover that extreme yang leads to yin and vice versa. Imagine your body in an extreme yang position (for example, your arms pushed forward as far as they will go, and your limbs extended and locked). You will reach a point at which you just can't push your arms out any further or make your leg any more locked. At this point your body becomes weak and is forced to relax – so it naturally goes back to a yin position. You can see this represented visually in the yin yang symbol. When the white (yang) side of the circle is at its most extreme point, yin starts to appear, and vice versa. The same is true in nature, as the sun (yang) reaches its highest point at midday, the light very gradually starts to fade until eventually it becomes dark (yin).

Sense the flow of chi

As you practise the Hand Form, remember that each tai chi posture is specifically designed to optimize the flow of chi through your meridians (see page 24). You can help this process by letting your breath sink to your lower abdomen, by tuning in to any tingling or warm sensations that you feel and by focusing your mind upon the movements of the Hand Form. The suggestions for visualizations I have included alongside some of the postures in Chapter 4 can help you get into a mentally focused state. So too can thinking about the titles of the postures and what they tell you about how you should practise each movement.

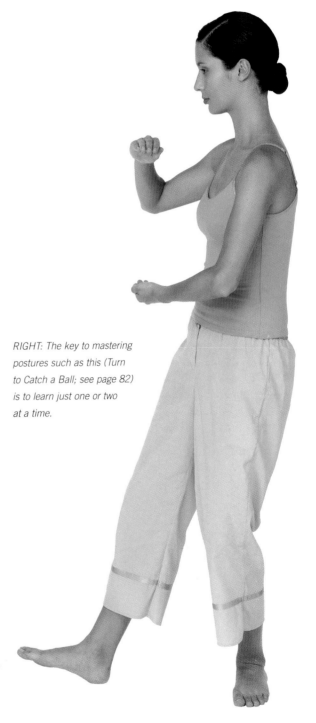

RIGHT: The key to mastering postures such as this (Turn to Catch a Ball; see page 82) is to learn just one or two at a time.

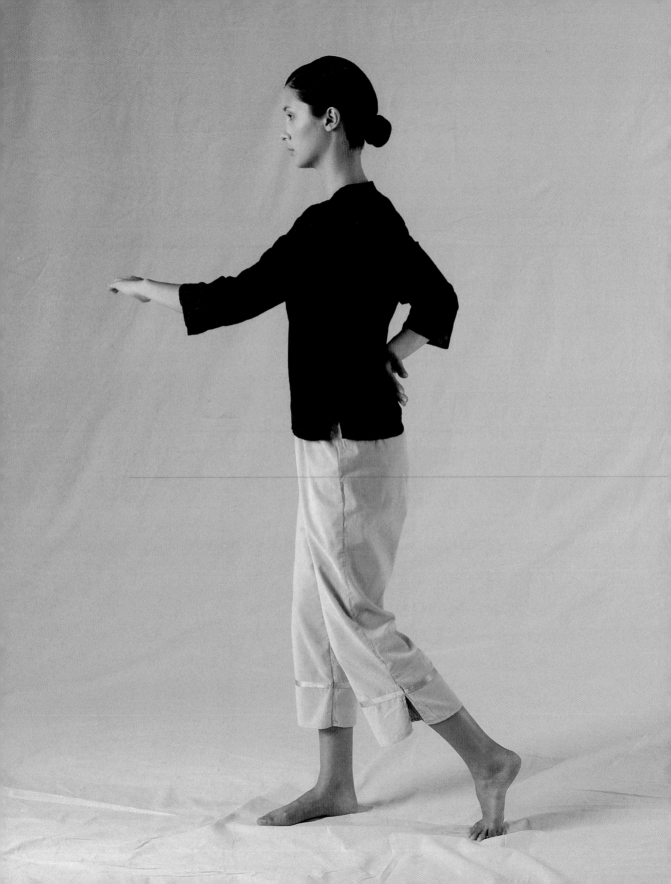

warm-up exercises

Before you practise the movements of tai chi in Chapter 4, it is important to prepare your body by making it loose and relaxed. The exercises in this chapter are all excellent ways of doing this. Many of the exercises come from the Chinese tradition of chi kung, which, literally translated, means "energy work". Chi kung exercises encourage chi (energy) to flow freely around your body – to give you a feeling of vitality – and they also release tension from your body, clear your mind and increase your mental focus. As well as being great ways of warming up for tai chi, the exercises in this chapter also make a stand-alone routine to practise at times when you simply want to unwind.

waist turn 1

This is a warm-up exercise that loosens your shoulders and waist.

This, in turn, stimulates energy flow throughout your body.

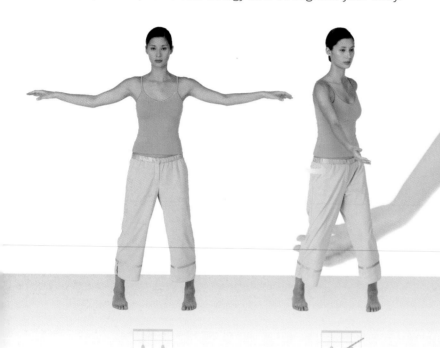

1 Start with your feet shoulder-distance apart and your arms extended at either side, shoulders down. Don't lock your arms.

✪ Keep your breath soft and natural throughout this exercise.

2 Turn at your waist toward the left. Let your arms drop as they follow the movement of your waist. Keep your feet facing forward.

◉ All the movement in this exercise comes from turning your waist. Keep both feet firmly in contact with the ground; this will help to open your pelvic area.

3 Continue turning until you reach your own comfortable limit. Let the centrifugal motion from your waist bring your arms up again. Now turn to the right. Keep turning in both directions.

◉ Visualize your shoulders dropping and your arms floating upward (don't use conscious muscular force).

waist turn 2

As you turn at the waist from one side to the other, your arms and hands slap against your body. Like the previous waist turn, this stimulates the flow of energy.

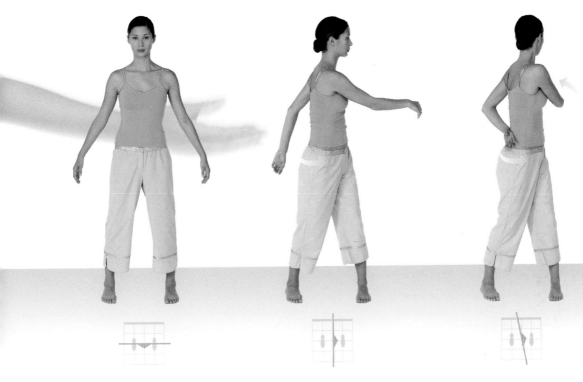

1 Start with your feet shoulder-distance apart and your arms gently extended by your sides.

2 Turn at your waist toward the left and allow your arms to follow the movement of your body in a loose, easy manner so they gently wrap around you.

3 When you've turned as far as you can, let your hands and arms gently slap your kidneys and chest to massage your body and stimulate energy flow. Keep turning in both directions.

forward and backward swings

This exercise trains you to transfer your weight forward and backward while maintaining a close connection to the ground and a light, open feeling in your upper body.

⊙ Have a sense of pushing through the sole of each foot as you move forward and back, and vice-versa. Let your arms be completely loose at the sides of your body – they will swing naturally as you transfer your weight. Be careful not to let your shoulders rise as your arms swing – let the weight of your arms keep your shoulders down.

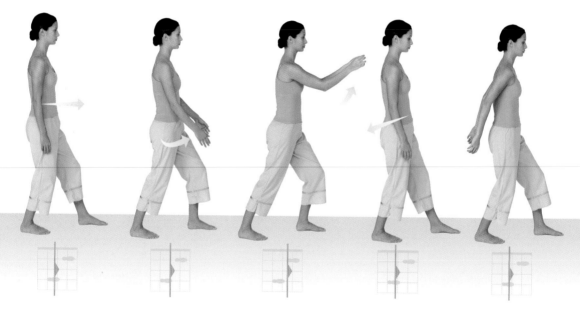

1 Start with your feet shoulder-distance apart and step forward with your left foot.

2 Carry your weight a little further forward. Let the forward motion of your body swing your arms upward.

3 Push off your right foot and transfer all your weight onto your left foot. Let your arms swing up as far as they will go.

4 Start to shift your weight backward until your weight is divided equally over each of your feet. Let your arms drop naturally to your sides.

5 Let your weight come fully onto your right foot. Let your arms swing behind you. Keep swinging forward and back in this way.

arm rotations

These arm rotations help to release blocked stress in your shoulders and upper body. Move slowly and carefully through this exercise, paying attention to any little aches or pains.

👁 Visualize your shoulder joint in its socket to get a sense of the full potential of this movement.

✪ If the movement feels tight or difficult, ease off and let your arm move in a wider arc at a distance from your side.

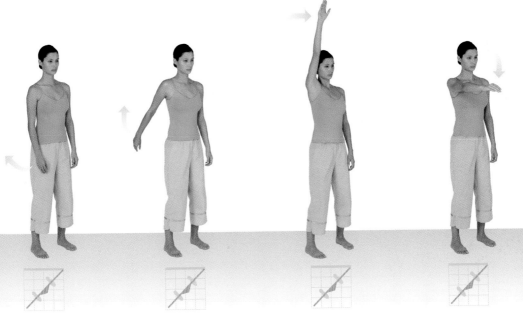

1 Stand with your feet shoulder-distance apart, your weight evenly distributed between your feet and your arms relaxed by your sides.

2 Slowly reach out behind you with your right arm and begin to lift it upward. Keep your shoulder down and your elbow slightly bent.

3 Let your arm pass your ear before bringing it to a fully vertical position. Point your hand upward.

4 Continue rolling your arm downward in a circle. Keep your shoulders relaxed. Do this rotation six times and then repeat with your left arm.

shoulder rotations

This exercise helps to clear your head. It also opens up your shoulders and upper body, areas where it's common for tension to accumulate. Start gently and don't force anything – take time to extend your physical limits.

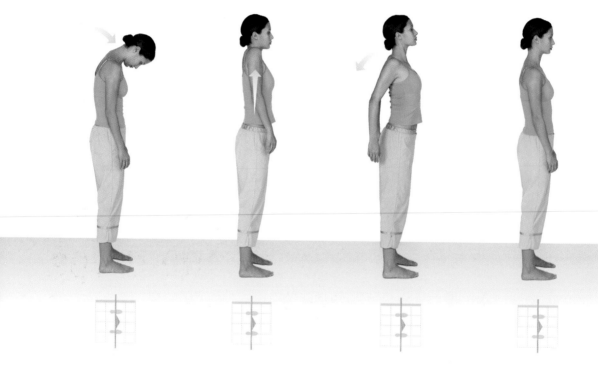

1 Start with your feet shoulder-distance apart, weight evenly distributed between your feet, and your knees soft. Drop your head forward until your chin is near your chest. Feel your upper back opening.

2 Slowly raise your head while pulling your shoulders up toward your ears. Gently inhale as you raise your shoulders.

3 Pull your shoulders backward and feel your chest opening as you slowly begin to exhale.

4 Still pulling backward and exhaling, lower and then relax your shoulders. Slowly drop your arms by your sides. Repeat the exercise, rotating your shoulders backward six times and forward six times.

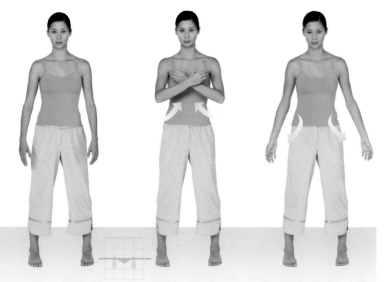

arm drops

This exercise is designed to loosen your shoulder joints and relax your arms. Imagine your arms are ropes and your hands are knots. Let the weight of the knots pull your shoulders down and connect you to the ground.

1 Start with your feet shoulder-distance apart, your toes pointing slightly inward and your arms by your sides.

2 Raise your arms and cross them in front of your body. Keep them light and open.

3 Let your arms drop back down to your sides. Do this six times.

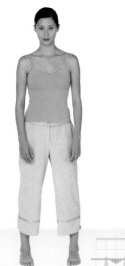

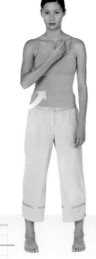

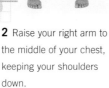

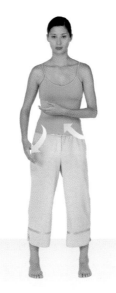

alternate arm drops

This variation of the previous exercise further loosens your shoulders and arms, and deepens your connection to the ground. Imagine each arm swinging like a pendulum. Create a natural rhythm.

1 Start with your feet shoulder-distance apart, your toes pointing slightly inward and your arms by your sides.

2 Raise your right arm to the middle of your chest, keeping your shoulders down.

3 Drop your right arm and raise your left one to the same position. Keep raising and dropping each arm.

limb-loosening exercises

This exercise loosens your arms and knee joints, and helps to increase your stability while standing on one leg.

1 Raise your left knee a little to gently rest your toes on the ground. Raise your arms in front of your body and loosely cross your hands.

2 Raise your left knee so that your foot comes off the ground. Slightly bend the knee of your right leg and keep your centre of gravity low. Raise your crossed hands to chest height.

3 Snap your left leg out from the knee as if you're kicking a ball. Drop your arms in front of you – feel them releasing from the shoulders and elbows. As you release your arms and leg, feel the strength of your connection with the earth through your right leg. Repeat with the other leg.

kidney strokes

This gentle exercise is useful if you have discomfort or tension in your kidney area, as it gently warms, softens and relaxes this part of your body.

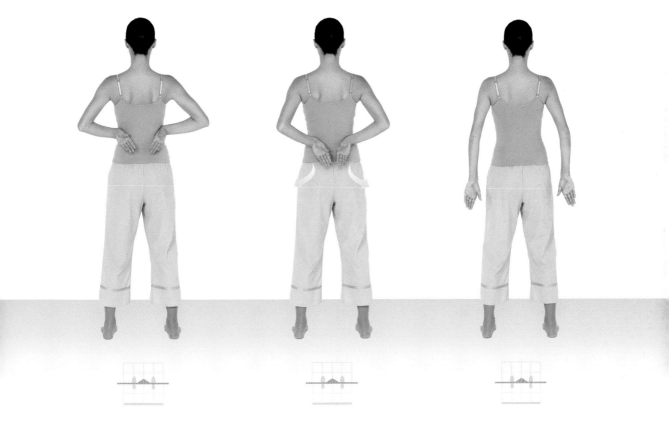

1 Place the backs of both wrists against the middle of your back, either side of your spine.

2 Press the backs of your wrists firmly against your back as you gently sweep them down and in toward your kidneys.

3 Repeat the exercise until you feel warmth in your lower back.

☯ Cheng Man Ching recommended 49 repetitions of this exercise every morning, before beginning daily tai chi practice.

lift hands

This exercise is similar to the first movement of the Hand Form (see Chapter 4). It is good for calming the mind, and it helps to settle the liver chi, which can become overactive, causing you to lose your composure.

The chi kung exercises that follow on pages 60–73 are similar to tai chi postures, but are practised as individual movements rather than part of a longer, flowing sequence. They are easy to learn and they act as a good complement to the tai chi Form. They can be learned relatively quickly and you should start to feel the benefits almost immediately.

☯ Keep your shoulders down and a sense of openness under your arms.

☯ Breathe softly and naturally, in time with your movements.

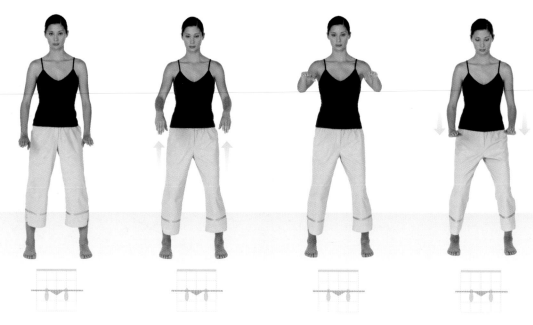

1 Stand with your feet shoulder-distance apart and your arms open by your sides. Begin to lift your hands.

2 Slowly lift your arms – imagine there is a thread at the backs of your wrists pulling them up.

3 Gently breathe in and raise your arms so they are roughly horizontal to the ground. Keep your palms relaxed.

4 Slowly lower your arms while bending your knees and sinking your weight. Breathe out and relax your arms. Repeat the exercise six times.

opening the chest

This exercise creates a feeling of freedom and expansiveness in your upper body. Imagine that you are manipulating a ball of energy between your palms.

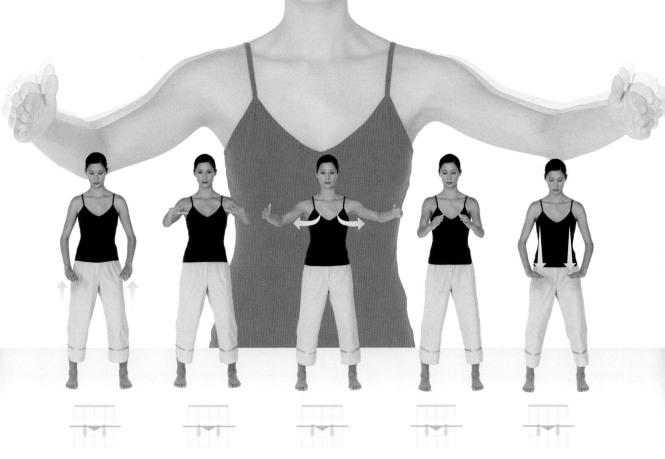

1 Stand with your feet shoulder-distance apart and your arms relaxed and open. Slowly begin to raise your arms.

2 Keep raising your arms until they are in front of you at chest-height, palms facing down.

3 As you breathe out, move your arms to the sides, parallel to the ground. Turn both palms to face inward.

4 Breathe in and bring your palms in toward each other as if you are holding a small ball at your chest.

5 Breathe out, lower your arms, palms facing down. Let your weight sink. Repeat the exercise six times.

punch tiger's ears

This exercise opens your upper body, increases the flow of energy in the heart and lung meridians and helps you to focus your mind.

⊘ Try not to raise your shoulders when you bring your arms up for the punch. When leaning forward, keep your spine aligned and your knee behind your toes.

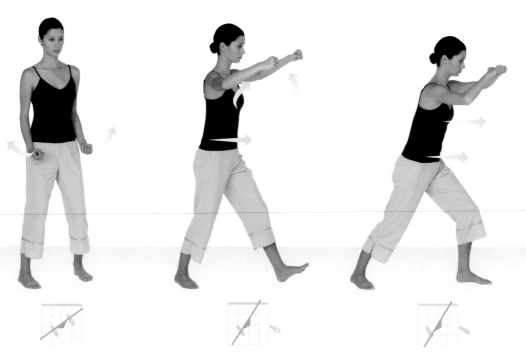

1 Stand with your feet facing forward, shoulder-width apart. Keep your arms by your sides with your hands curled into soft fists on either side of your hips.

2 As you breathe in, step forward and gently place your left heel on the ground. Bring your arms up in a circular movement so your fists are level with your face.

3 As you breathe out, transfer your weight almost fully forward on to your left foot. Bring your fists together in front of you as if punching the ears of an imaginary opponent. Return to the starting position and repeat, this time stepping forward with your right foot.

touch the sea, look at the sky

This exercise increases the flow of energy in the heart and lung meridians, and helps to combat depression and melancholy by opening your upper body.

⊕ Keep your hands, fingers and upper body light and open. Maintain a low centre of gravity as you lean forward. Try not to lift your shoulders in the third position.

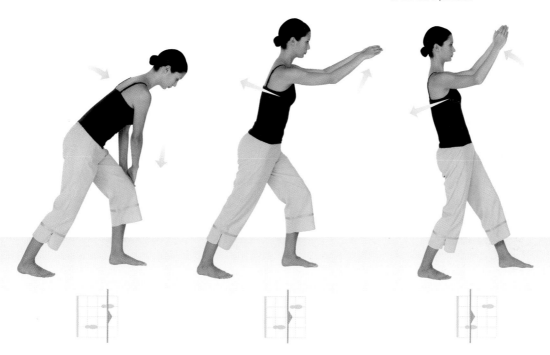

1 Start with your left foot forward. Bend forward keeping your spine aligned. Place your hands one on top of the other at the level of your left knee.

2 Slowly shift your weight back onto your right leg and bring your spine into an upright position. Raise your arms in front of you, keeping them slightly bent.

3 Move your weight back as far as you can without losing stability. Raise your arms above your head and out to the sides. Return to the starting position, but this time with your right foot forward. Repeat the exercise.

lion plays with ball

This exercise improves your mental focus, helps to open your upper body and increases your energy flow. It also exercises the muscles in the area of your heart.

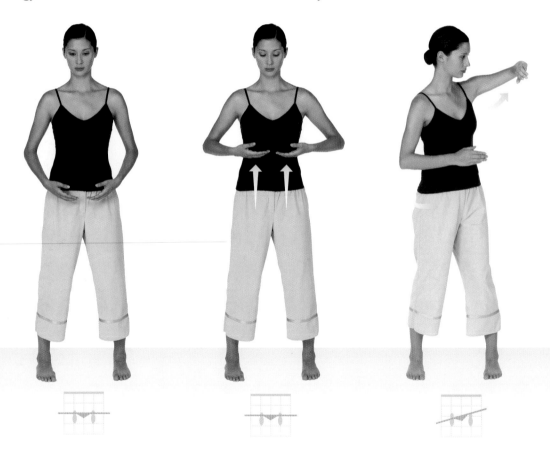

1 Start with your feet shoulder-distance apart and your palms facing upward as if you are holding a ball.

2 Bring your hands to the middle of your upper body. Keep your palms facing upward.

3 Start to turn to the left from your waist. Turn your right palm in to face your body and raise your left hand, palm facing out.

☯ Keep your shoulders down when you lift
your arms. When you turn, focus on turning
from your waist, and on keeping your back
aligned. When you push outward, keep your
hands soft and relaxed.

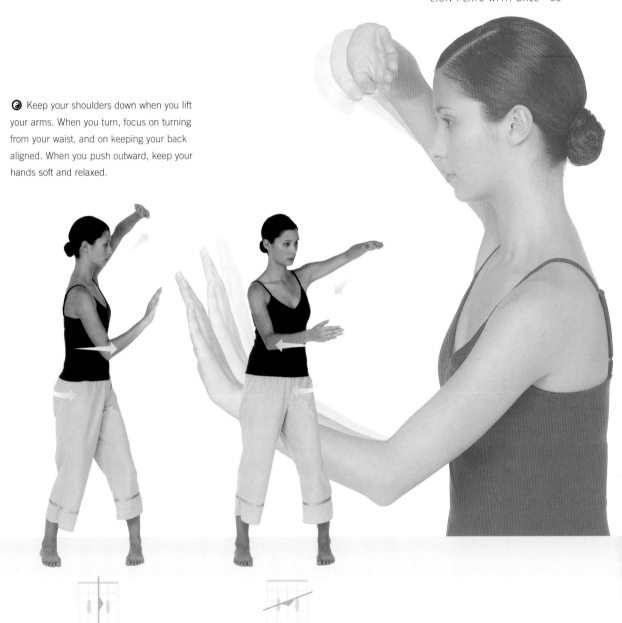

4 Keep turning from your waist. Raise
your left hand just above your head,
palm facing up. Move your right arm
forward at chest height as if you are
pushing a ball outward.

5 Turn back to face the front. Slowly
bring your arms back down to the starting
position (step 1). Repeat steps 2–5 on
the other side of your body.

crossing the wide blue ocean

This exercise is good for the healthy functioning of your bladder and kidneys because of its watery imagery. It also helps to clear tension and anxiety.

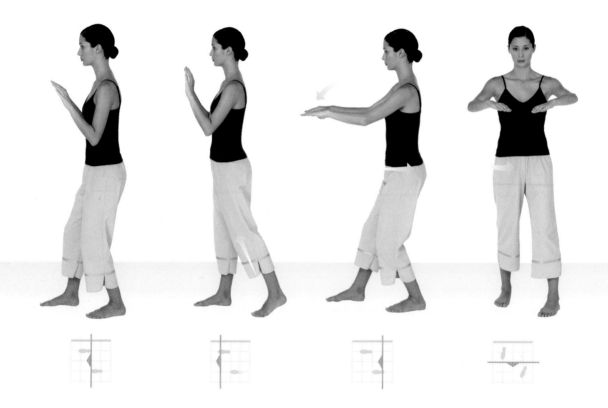

1 Start with your weight on your left foot. Bend your arms so that your forearms are close to your body, palms facing outward in preparation for pushing forward. Breathe in.

2 Breathe out and, pushing off from your left foot, transfer your weight upward and then forward onto your right foot. Push forward with your arms.

3 Shift your weight back on to your left foot and allow your arms to lengthen out in front of you as if they are lying on the surface of the sea. Breathe out as you transfer your weight.

4 Still breathing out, turn at your waist toward the left. Keep your shoulders down and your arms open.

When you push forward, keep your upper body light and open – this will prevent you over-balancing. Turn from your waist rather than your upper body, and take care not to raise your shoulders.

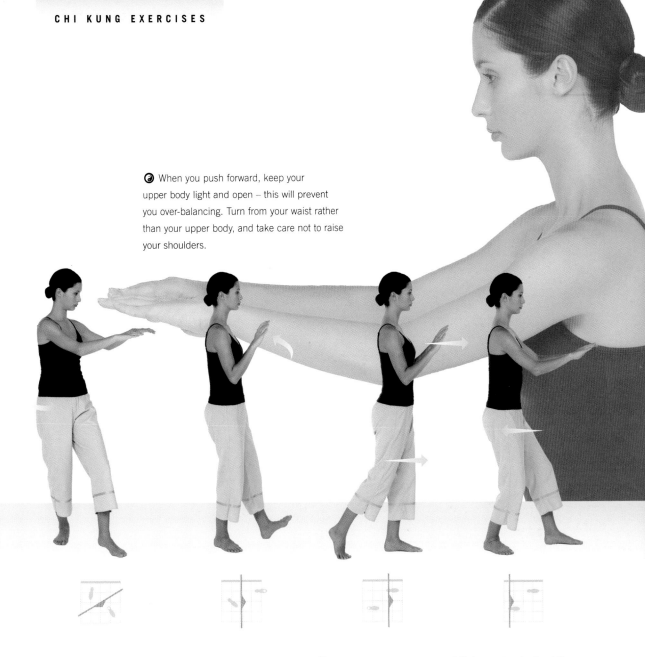

5 Keep turning from your waist until your body faces the left side.

6 As you breathe in, shift your weight onto your right foot while bringing your arms closer in to your body.

7 As you breathe out, push forward with your arms and transfer your weight onto your left foot.

8 As you breathe in, shift your weight back on to your right foot and allow your arms to lengthen out in front of you.

yinjinjing exercises

Perform these simple exercises as strongly as you can. You should feel the energy surging through your body almost immediately.

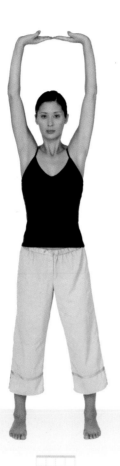

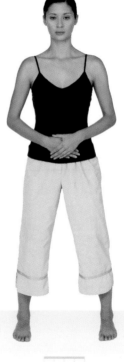

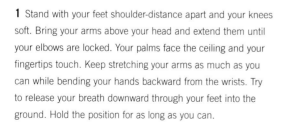

1 Stand with your feet shoulder-distance apart and your knees soft. Bring your arms above your head and extend them until your elbows are locked. Your palms face the ceiling and your fingertips touch. Keep stretching your arms as much as you can while bending your hands backward from the wrists. Try to release your breath downward through your feet into the ground. Hold the position for as long as you can.

2 When you have to release your arms, slowly lower them and bring them to a resting position in which your palms rest, one on top of the other, on your lower abdomen. Spend a few moments connecting with your breath in your lower abdomen until it settles and becomes calm.

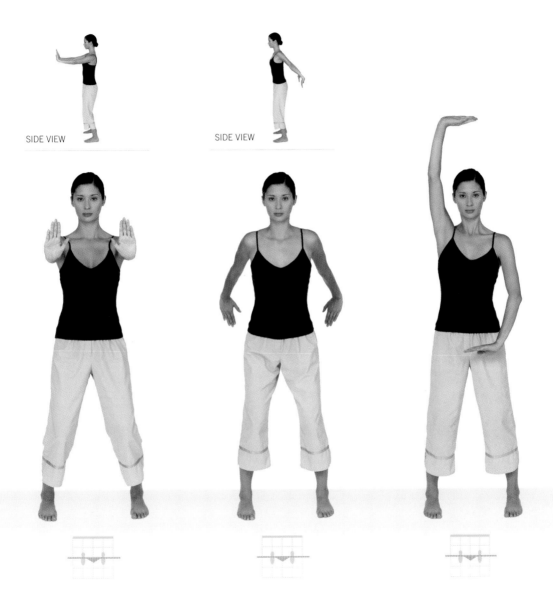

SIDE VIEW

SIDE VIEW

3 Stand with your feet shoulder-distance apart and your knees soft. Push your arms in front of you, parallel to the floor, palms facing forward. Stretch as far as you can while pulling your fingers back toward your body. Hold the stretch for as long as you can. Then return to step 2.

4 Stand with your feet shoulder-distance apart and your knees soft. Push your arms out behind you. Stretch as far as you can while pulling your fingers back toward your body. When you can't hold the stretch any longer, bring your palms to rest on your abdomen as in step 2.

5 Stand with your feet shoulder-distance apart and your knees soft. Stretch one hand above your head, palm facing up. Keep your other hand at waist-height, palm down. Hold the stretch for as long as you can and then slowly return to step 2. Now repeat with your other arm raised.

zhan zhuang postures

Standing postures create a strong connection to the energies of earth below and the heavens above. They promote good bodily alignment and relaxation. Stand in these positions for 1 or 2 minutes at first, and build up to 5 or more minutes.

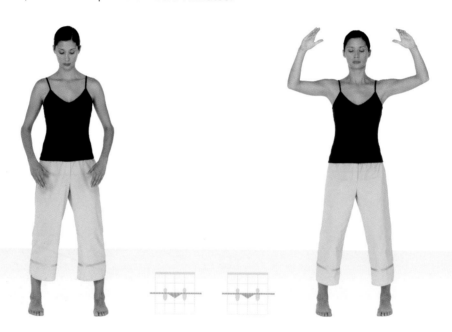

PREPARATION POSTURE

You can do this meditative exercise by itself or before you do the tai chi. Stand with your feet shoulder-distance apart, your knees soft, your shoulders down, your elbows unlocked and your hands soft and open. Close your eyes or softly focus on the far distance. Let tension flow out of you. Feel warmth gather at the centre of your palms.

◉ Imagine your body is an egg timer. Slowly let the sand empty from your head, through your body and into the ground.

HOLDING A BALL ABOVE YOUR HEAD

This posture stimulates the flow of energy in your upper body and helps to focus your mind. Stand with your feet shoulder-distance apart, your knees soft, your shoulders down, your elbows unlocked and your hands soft and open. Hold your arms above your head, palms facing forward. Close your eyes and connect your tongue to your upper palate, just behind your teeth. Observe whether your weight shifts back or forward – try to keep your body aligned. Sense how your feet connect to the ground through your Yongquan points (see page 26).

HOLDING A CHI BALL

This is a calming posture. Stand with your feet shoulder-distance apart, your knees soft, your shoulders down, your elbows unlocked and your hands soft and open. Raise your arms to chest height with your palms facing your body. Close your eyes and connect your tongue to your upper palate, just behind your top teeth. Notice whether your weight shifts forward or back – try to keep your body aligned. Be aware of the connection of your feet to the ground through your Yongquan points.

✪ Let your breath relax into your lower abdomen.

STANDING IN A STREAM

This posture helps you to build stamina and internal strength. Stand with your feet shoulder-distance apart, your knees soft, your shoulders down, your elbows unlocked and your hands soft and open. Hold your arms out by your sides at waist height, palms down, as if you are about to walk a tightrope. Close your eyes and connect your tongue to your upper palate, just behind your teeth. Observe whether your weight shifts forward or back – try keep your body aligned. Be aware of the connection of your feet to the ground through your Yongquan points.

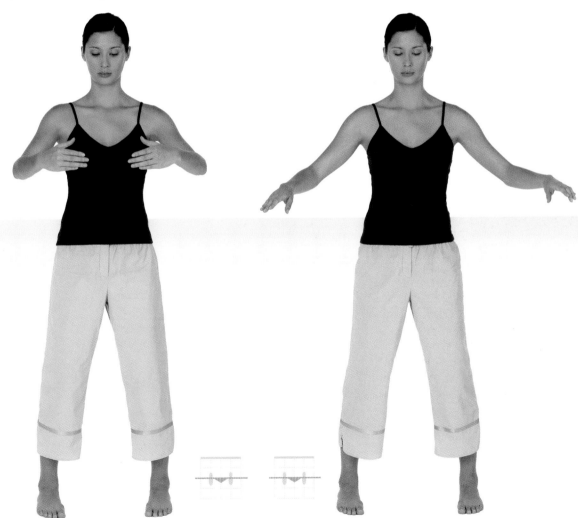

sau gong

This is a good exercise to end your warm-up session because it gathers and stores chi in your lower dantien (see page 27). Sau Gong means "collecting the chi".

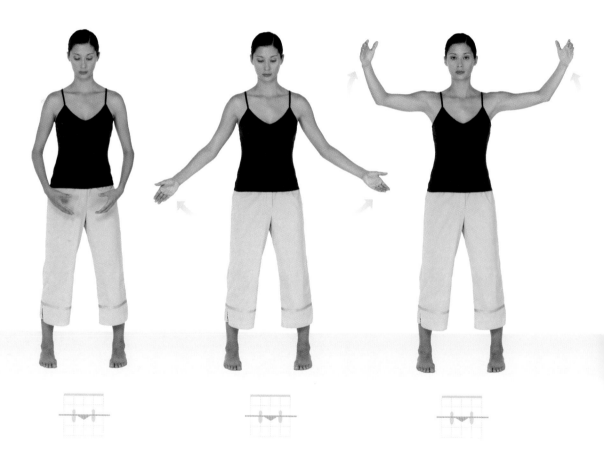

1 Start with your feet shoulder-distance apart and your palms softly open and facing each other.

2 Turn your palms to face up, and slowly raise your arms on either side of your body while breathing in.

3 Let your arms reach upward. Keep your shoulders down and your breathing relaxed and soft.

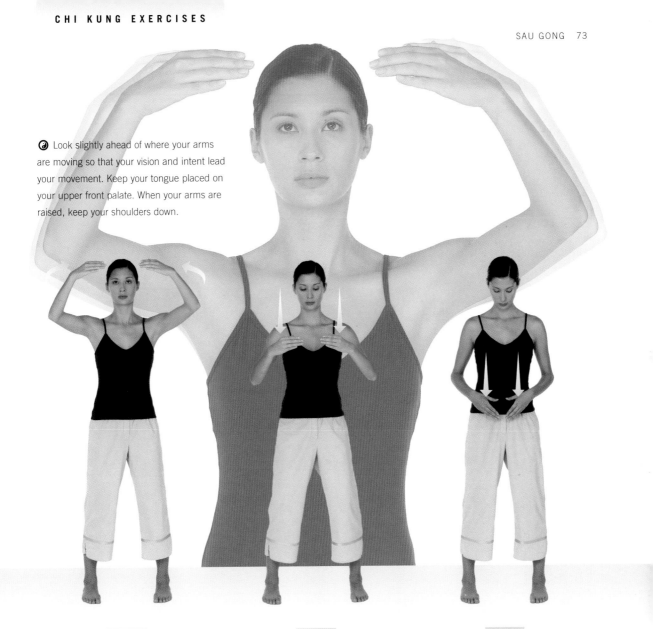

☯ Look slightly ahead of where your arms are moving so that your vision and intent lead your movement. Keep your tongue placed on your upper front palate. When your arms are raised, keep your shoulders down.

4 Turn your palms to face down as you slowly breathe out and lower your arms in front of your face and body.

5 Continue to breathe out as you lower your arms. Imagine that you are pushing energy down to your lower abdomen.

6 Let your palms face your lower dantien so that your Laogong points (see page 26) focus the chi to be stored in this area. Repeat this exercise six times.

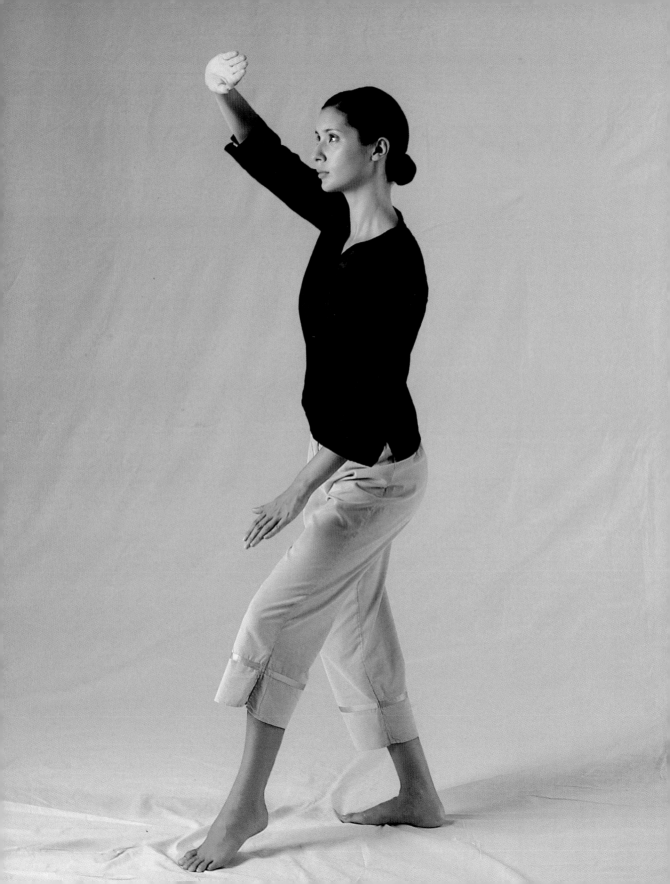

the movements of tai chi

This chapter contains a sequence of tai chi postures known as the Hand Form. It is a shortened version of the traditional tai chi Form and it was devised by Cheng Man Ching (see page 30).

Try not to be in a hurry to learn the postures in this chapter. It is better to spend 10 to 15 minutes working on two or three postures a day, rather than trying to do the whole sequence at once. Allow time for your mind to absorb information, rather than forcing the learning process. By continually repeating the movements with a calm, clear mind, each posture will work its way into a deep level of your consciousness.

When you are familiar with the sequence, work on moving smoothly and fluidly from one posture to the next. In time, you will be able to move seamlessly through the entire sequence from the Beginning Posture to Cross Hands and Close.

hand, arm, feet and leg positions

These are the correct positions for your hands, arms, feet and legs during the Hand Form (see pages 80–105). Look at the photographs below and try to keep them in your mind's eye – this will help you to replicate the positions during your tai chi practice.

hand and arm positions

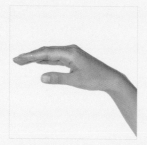

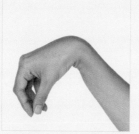

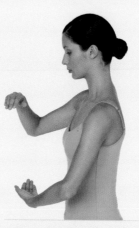

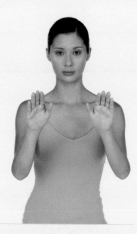

OPEN PALMS
This is the basic hand position that you should use during most of the Form, including the Push postures (see pages 96–7). Keep the inside of your palm soft, relaxed and slightly rounded inward, and the back of your hand relaxed with no tension in the tendons.

THE HOOK
Use this position during Single Whip (see pages 90–91). Let your hand drop downward from the wrist with all your fingers coming softly together, and your forefinger and second finger coming lightly into contact with your thumb.

CUPPED PALMS
Use this position in sequences such as Catch a Ball (see page 83). Your downward-facing palm is softly open as if you are warming your hand at a fire. Your upward-facing palm is curved so that you would be able to hold a small ball without gripping it.

PUSH
Use this position in the Push postures. Keep your elbows and shoulders down, your arms just inside the line of your body, a sense of openness under your arms and your palms relaxed and facing the centre of the chest of an imaginary opponent. The Push comes from the heel of your hands.

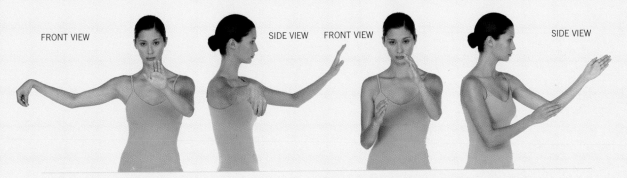

FRONT VIEW   SIDE VIEW   FRONT VIEW   SIDE VIEW

ARM POSITIONS FOR SINGLE WHIP (SEE PAGES 90–91)
Your left hand faces directly forward in line with the centre of
your body. Your elbow is down – keep a sense of openness
under your arm. Your right arm is stretched out to the side
with your elbow bent and relaxed and your shoulder down.
Your right hand is in a hook shape (see opposite).

☯ Your hand alignment is important in these two postures.

ARM POSITIONS FOR PLAY GUITAR (SEE PAGES 92–3)
Extend your arms so that they cover the central line of your
body; your left hand is in line with your nose (to protect your
face) and your right hand is opposite the inside of your left
elbow to create a fulcrum together with your arm when your
attacking arm comes forward. Keep your arms open and
relaxed and your shoulders and elbows down.

feet and leg positions

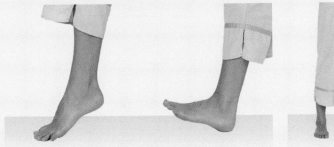 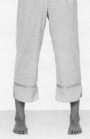

CAT STANCE
Use this in White Crane
Spreads Wings (see page 95)
and Step Up To Play Guitar
(see page 98). Keep your
weight on your back foot as
the toes of your front foot rest
on the ground. Imagine
dipping your toes in water.

HEEL ON GROUND, TOE UP
Use this in Play Guitar (see
pages 92–3). Keep almost all
of your weight on your back
foot. Rest gently on the heel of
your front foot as if you are
deciding whether or not to
transfer your weight forward.

SHOULDER-DISTANCE
APART, SIDE BY SIDE
This is a classic starting
position. Stand with your feet
shoulder-distance apart and
your toes pointing slightly
inward so that the outsides
of your feet are parallel.
Keep your knees in line with
your feet.

SHOULDER-DISTANCE
APART, ONE FOOT FORWARD
Use this throughout the Form.
Stand with your feet shoulder-
distance apart, with your front
knee bent and your front foot
forward and carrying 70 per
cent of your weight. Turn your
back foot to a 45-degree angle
with your front foot.

basic stepping exercise

☯ You can practise these steps as a calming meditative exercise.

☯ Keep your breath relaxed and your eyes softly focused.

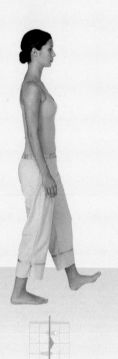

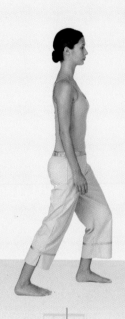

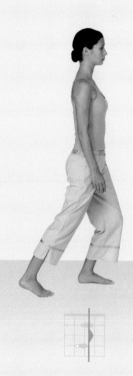

THE FIRST STEP

Place your left heel gently on the ground in front of you (a comfortable distance forward). Your toes should be facing forward. Keep your centre of gravity low and your upper body light and open. Face forward and softly focus straight ahead in the far distance. Make sure that both your knees are bent, particularly your left knee.

PLACING THE LEFT FOOT

Gradually allow the sole of your left foot to come to the ground but don't put any weight on it. Keep your upper body light and open – your body will naturally find a comfortable alignment and this will prevent you leaning forward. Keep your right leg soft around the knee joint. Let your arms hang loosely by your sides, with space under your arms.

TRANSFERRING THE WEIGHT

Gently raise the heel of your right foot and transfer your weight onto your left foot. Don't raise your knees. Keeping your gravity low will help you establish a strong connection to the ground and maintain a comfortable balance. Let your breath settle quietly in your lower abdomen – this also helps to keep your centre of gravity low.

Stepping from one posture to another is an integral aspect of tai chi. A good transition between postures means that you transfer your weight smoothly without disturbing the equilibrium of your body. It's common for students to concentrate on getting the individual postures right, but to forget about doing the connecting movements correctly. This stepping exercise is worth practising by itself – a firm, stable footing will serve you well throughout your training.

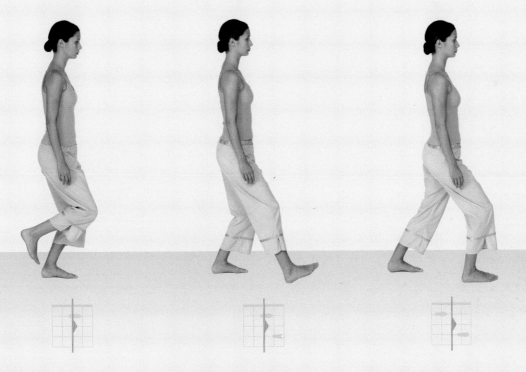

THE SECOND STEP
Keep your centre of gravity low on your left foot and start to pull your right foot through in preparation for stepping forward. To keep your balance stable, avoid raising your right knee.

PLACING THE RIGHT HEEL
Gently place your right heel on the ground with your toes facing forward. Keep your back knee and your centre of gravity low. Centre your breath in your lower abdomen – this will help you relax and connect to the exercise.

PLACING THE RIGHT FOOT
Slowly let the whole of your front foot rest on the ground in preparation for transferring your weight forward. Try to be aware of each part of your foot making contact with the ground.

beginning posture

Despite its apparent simplicity, the Beginning Posture is the most important posture in the Hand Form – this is where you prepare yourself for the sequence ahead.

Stand with your feet shoulder-distance apart and your toes pointing slightly inward so that the outsides of your feet are parallel. Soften your knees and feel your connection with the ground through the Yongquan point (see page 26) in the centre of the front of the soles of your feet. Tuck in your hips slightly – as though you are sitting on a high stool – to bring your back into alignment. Hollow your chest a little and tuck your chin in – this releases strain from the back of your neck. Connect your tongue to your upper palate and allow your breath to sink slowly to your lower abdomen. Spend a few minutes allowing your body and mind to relax and settle. Connect to the ground from your waist down and be light and open to the heavens from your waist up.

👁 Imagine that you have tennis balls resting in your armpits – this creates openness in your arms.

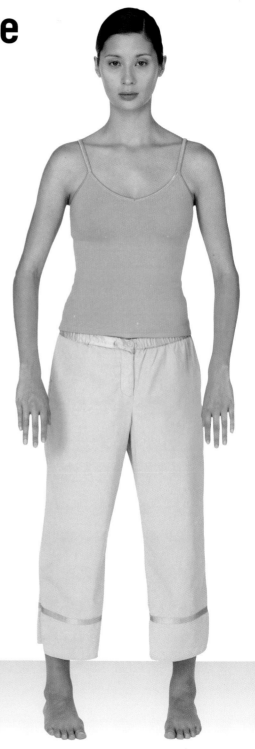

lift hands and lower hands and sink

◉ Imagine your wrists are tied to two balloons that are floating upward. Your elbows are hung with weights that keep them down as your arms rise.

◉ Imagine you are gently pressing down a balloon under each palm. As you sink, visualize a pole against your back – this will prevent you from leaning forward or backward.

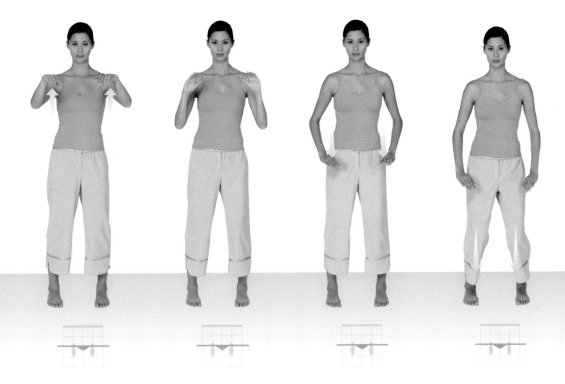

LIFT HANDS

Let your arms rise upward until they are almost at shoulder height. Keep your hands soft and relaxed, and a sense of openness under your arms. Try to feel the air moving around your arms. Now bend your arms and draw your hands toward your body. Don't let your shoulders rise. Look forward with a soft focus. Centre your attention on the tips of your fingers.

LOWER HANDS AND SINK

Lower your arms until your palms are just below your hips. At the same time, slowly start to sink by bending your knees – but don't let your knees extend beyond your toes. Gaze forward and concentrate on the point at the centre of your palms – the Laogong point. Hold your palms softly open, as if you are warming your hands at a fire below.

turn to catch a ball

Let all of your body weight come onto your left foot while you turn 90 degrees to your right. Let this movement originate from your waist, and keep your arms soft and relaxed. Allow your right arm to rise so that the centre of your wrist aligns with the middle of your upper chest, palm facing downward. Bring your left arm, palm facing upward, to waist height so that it is aligned with your right hand. Turn your head with your body. Gaze ahead.

👁 Imagine you are holding a light ball between your hands. Feel a connection between the centres of both of your palms.

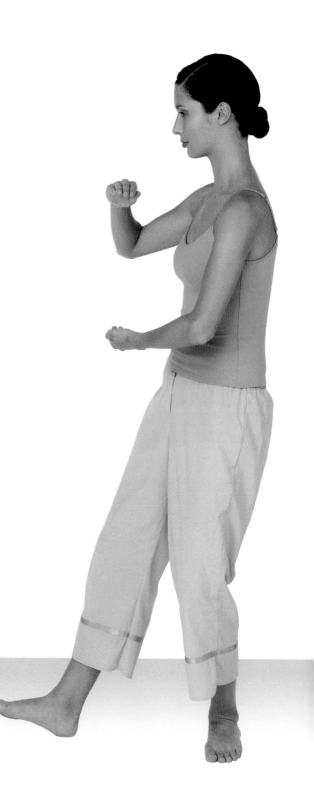

catch a ball

Slowly shift 70 per cent of your weight onto your right foot. This weight transfer should come from low down in your body – let your upper body stay light and open. Keep a sense of openness under your arms and keep your palms soft and relaxed, as if you are holding a light ball or a balloon. Relax your stomach and keep your breathing focused in your lower abdomen.

◉ As you move your weight onto your right foot, imagine that someone is gently pushing you forward by pressing on your lower back.

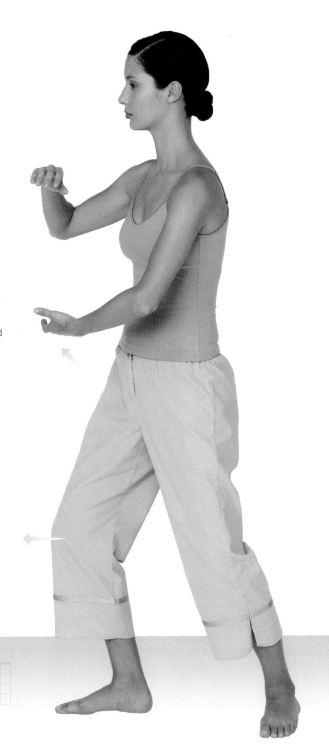

prepare to ward-off left, brush sparrow's tail

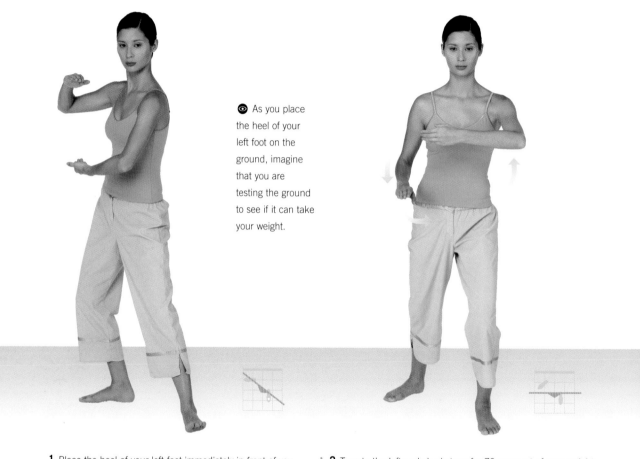

👁 As you place the heel of your left foot on the ground, imagine that you are testing the ground to see if it can take your weight.

1 Place the heel of your left foot immediately in front of you. Your feet should be shoulder-distance apart. Gaze in the direction you are about to go. Keep your arms a comfortable, open distance from your body, and your palms soft and facing each other.

2 Turn to the left and slowly transfer 70 per cent of your weight onto your left foot. Check your feet are still shoulder-distance apart. As you transfer your weight, turn your right foot, from the heel. Bring your left wrist in line with the centre of your upper chest and lower your right arm with your palm facing downward. Keep both hands relaxed and open. Check that your left foot, pelvis and head are all facing the same direction.

prepare to ward-off right, brush sparrow's tail

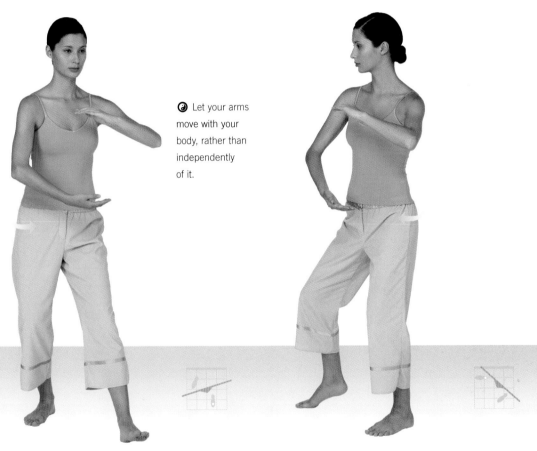

☯ Let your arms move with your body, rather than independently of it.

1 Shift your weight back onto your right foot and turn to your left. Let the movement come from your waist and keep the rest of your body soft and light. Feel a sense of connection to the ground through your right foot.

2 Shift your weight back onto your left foot while slowly turning your body to your right. Step forward with your right foot, being careful not to transfer your weight. Allow your gaze to turn toward your right in preparation for the next movement.

ward-off right

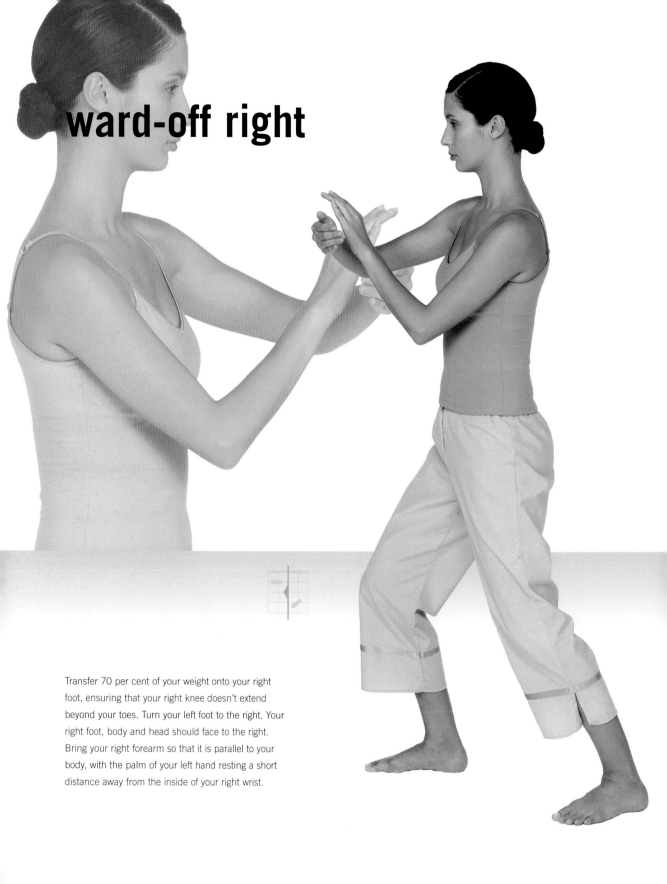

Transfer 70 per cent of your weight onto your right foot, ensuring that your right knee doesn't extend beyond your toes. Turn your left foot to the right. Your right foot, body and head should face to the right. Bring your right forearm so that it is parallel to your body, with the palm of your left hand resting a short distance away from the inside of your right wrist.

roll back

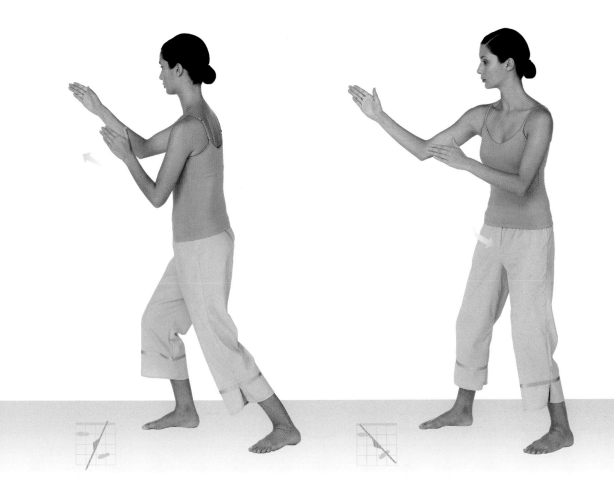

1 Turn your waist 45 degrees to the right, allowing your arms to turn with your body. Bring your right hand to point forward and the palm of your left hand to face the inside of your right elbow. Bring 80 per cent of your weight onto your right foot. Keep the area under your arms open and relaxed, and your palms soft. Concentrate on the area forward of your right hand.

2 Turn from your waist toward the left, letting your arms turn with you so they stay opposite the centre of your body. As you turn, slowly shift 70 per cent of your weight back onto your left foot. Keep your arms open and extended. Keep your right foot facing forward and your left foot at an angle of 45 degrees.

press 1 and 2

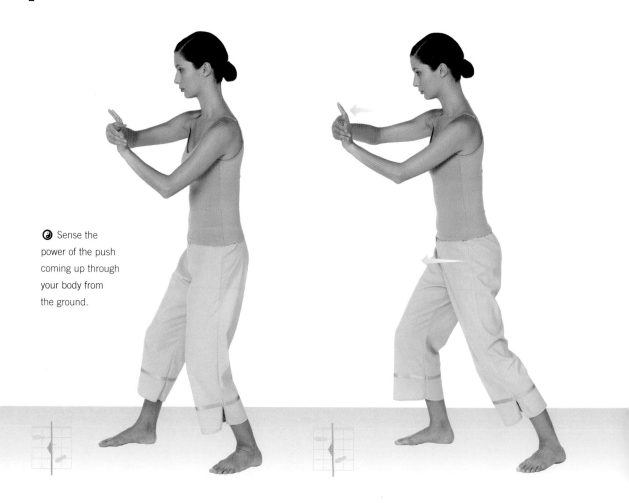

☯ Sense the power of the push coming up through your body from the ground.

1 Turn from your waist to face the right. Bring your right forearm parallel to your chest, a reasonable distance away. Rest the heel of your left hand on the inside of your right wrist. Keep your energy connected to the ground as you prepare to move forward from your left foot.

2 Shift 70 per cent of your weight forward onto your right foot, ensuring that your right knee stays behind your toes. Press forward – the Press starts in your back leg and comes through your left hand and into your right wrist. Keep your arms and hands soft. Focus ahead in the direction of the Press.

split and retract, and push

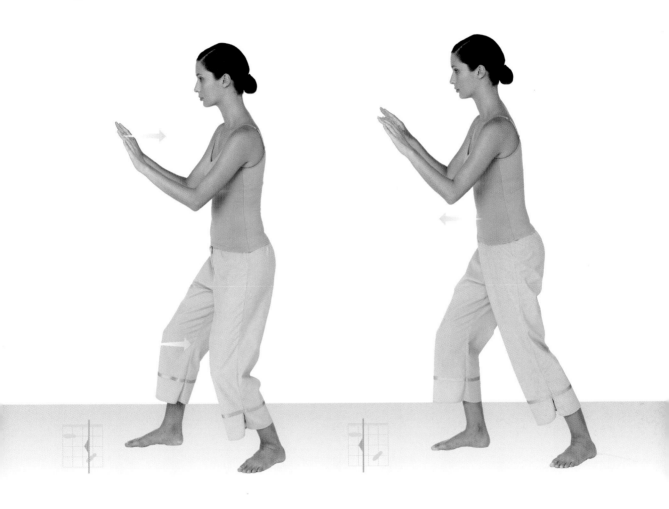

1 Bring your arms shoulder-distance apart with your elbows down and the palms of your hands facing forward. Slowly shift 70 per cent of your weight onto your left foot. Relax your stomach and keep your breath in your lower abdomen.

2 Shift 70 per cent of your weight forward onto your right foot and let your palms come forward with your body to push into the centre of the chest of an imaginary opponent. The strength of the Push comes through your back foot, up your legs, through your arms and into your hands, which should remain soft and relaxed. Keep your shoulders down and avoid over-extending your arms or upper body.

single whip

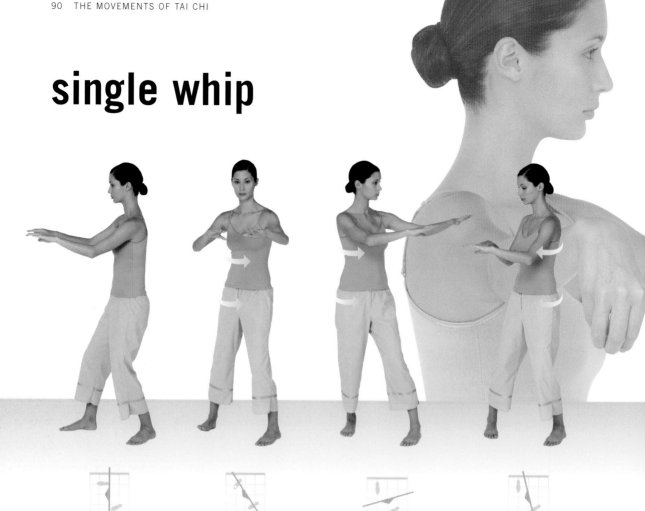

1 Slowly transfer your weight back onto your left foot. Allow your arms to lengthen without getting locked at the elbow. Don't lock your right knee or lean backward. Keep your shoulders down and your breath relaxed in your lower abdomen.

2 Your weight should now be completely on your left foot. Turn your right foot 90 degrees toward the front while turning at your waist to face forward. Focus in front as you turn. Keep your arms open, soft and parallel to the floor, and your shoulders down.

3 Keep turning until you have moved through 180 degrees to face the left. Keep your head in alignment with your spine, and keep a sense of lightness and openness in your upper body.

4 With your weight still on your left foot, turn 180 degrees back toward your right. Keep your arms open and soft, and parallel to the floor, and your shoulders down. Look straight ahead.

⊙ Imagine you are holding a pinch of salt between the fingers and thumb of your right hand.

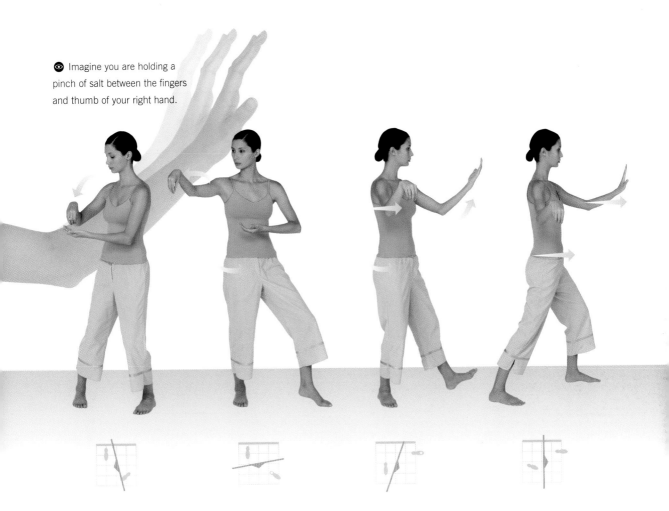

5 Bring your left hand in front of you at waist level, palm facing up. Allow your right hand to rest just above it. Bring the fingers and thumb of your right hand together. Keep your weight on your left foot as you prepare to turn and shift your weight to the left.

6 As you turn to the left, transfer your weight to your right foot. Turn the ball of your left foot so that it faces to the left. Allow your right arm to extend outward by your side – don't fully extend your elbow and keep your shoulder down. Keep your left arm slightly out from your body, with your palm facing up at waist height.

7 Step a shoulder-width to your left and gently place your left heel on the ground. Align your head, pelvis, knee and toes and face to the left. Raise your left arm in front of your body, palm facing inward.

8 Start to transfer your weight onto your left foot. Bring your left hand in line with the centre of your body, palm extending forward. As you transfer your weight, turn your right foot by 45 degrees. Finish the posture with 70 per cent of your weight on your left foot. Keep your left knee just behind your left toes.

play guitar

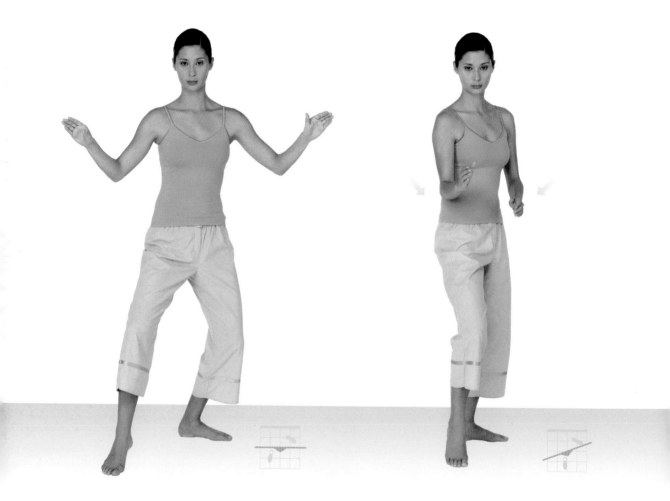

1 Shift more of your weight onto your left foot and turn your right foot to the right. Open your arms to each side, palms facing forward. Don't let your shoulders rise. Keep your breath relaxed. Focus straight ahead.

2 Keep focusing ahead as you turn your body slightly to the left. Bring your arms closer together – elbows near your waist and shoulders down – as if in preparation for an on-coming attack. Extend your right arm forward. Touch the ground with the toes of your right foot and take most of your weight on your left foot.

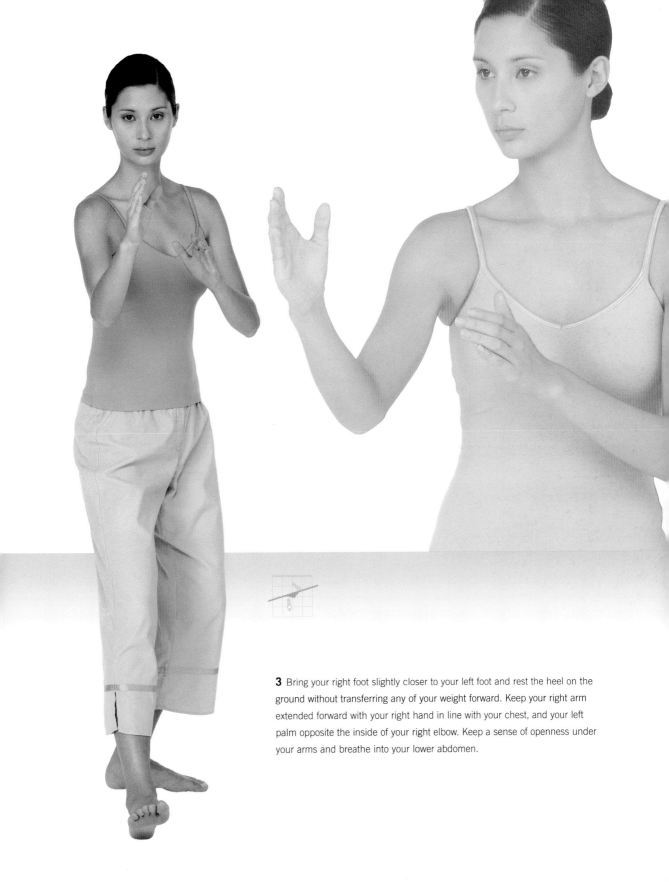

3 Bring your right foot slightly closer to your left foot and rest the heel on the ground without transferring any of your weight forward. Keep your right arm extended forward with your right hand in line with your chest, and your left palm opposite the inside of your right elbow. Keep a sense of openness under your arms and breathe into your lower abdomen.

shoulder stroke 1 and 2

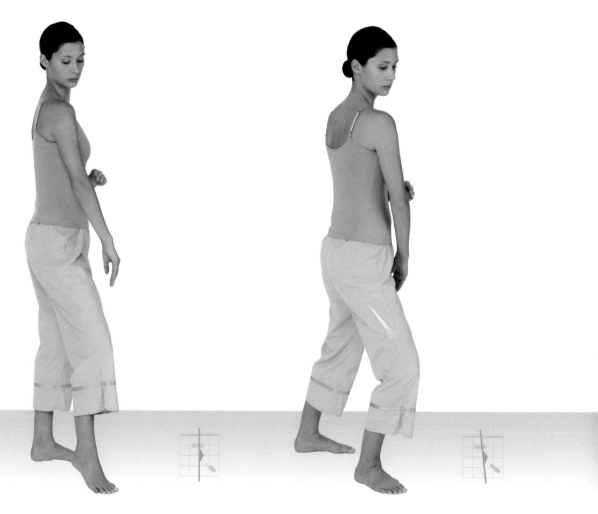

1 Turn to the left. Step forward with your right foot, just resting your toes on the ground without transferring your weight forward. Drop your right arm so your right palm faces your groin. Bring your left palm to face the inside of your right elbow.

2 Turn your body slightly more to the left. Place your right heel on the ground and start to transfer your weight forward, ensuring your right shoulder, knee and toes are facing in the same direction. Keep a sense of openness and space under your arms. Keep your right elbow directly underneath your shoulder. Finish with 70 per cent of your weight on your right foot.

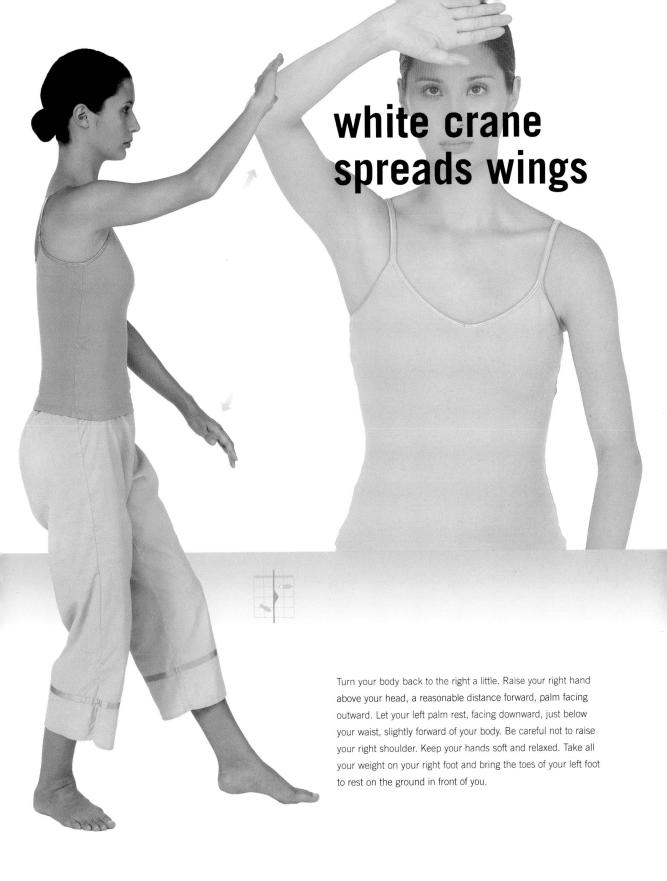

white crane
spreads wings

Turn your body back to the right a little. Raise your right hand above your head, a reasonable distance forward, palm facing outward. Let your left palm rest, facing downward, just below your waist, slightly forward of your body. Be careful not to raise your right shoulder. Keep your hands soft and relaxed. Take all your weight on your right foot and bring the toes of your left foot to rest on the ground in front of you.

brush left knee and push

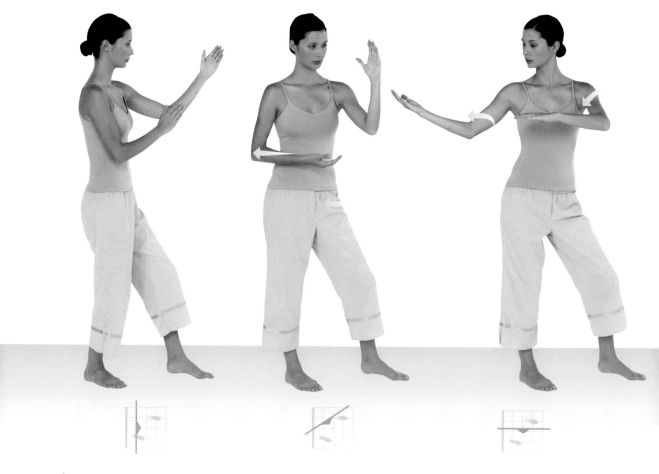

1 Face toward the left. Bring your left arm up so your left hand is in line with your nose. Your right hand should rest just inside your left elbow. Keep all your weight on your right foot, your shoulders down and your breathing relaxed in your lower abdomen.

2 Turn from your waist toward the right. Bring your right forearm horizontally in front of your body, palm facing up.

☯ Keep a sense of openness under your arms.

3 Lengthen your right arm gently out to the side without stretching or locking it. Fold your left arm horizontally in front of your body, palm facing down. Your left arm should be the same distance from your body as your elbow is from your shoulder. Keep your shoulders down and your breathing relaxed in your lower abdomen. Turn your head to the right.

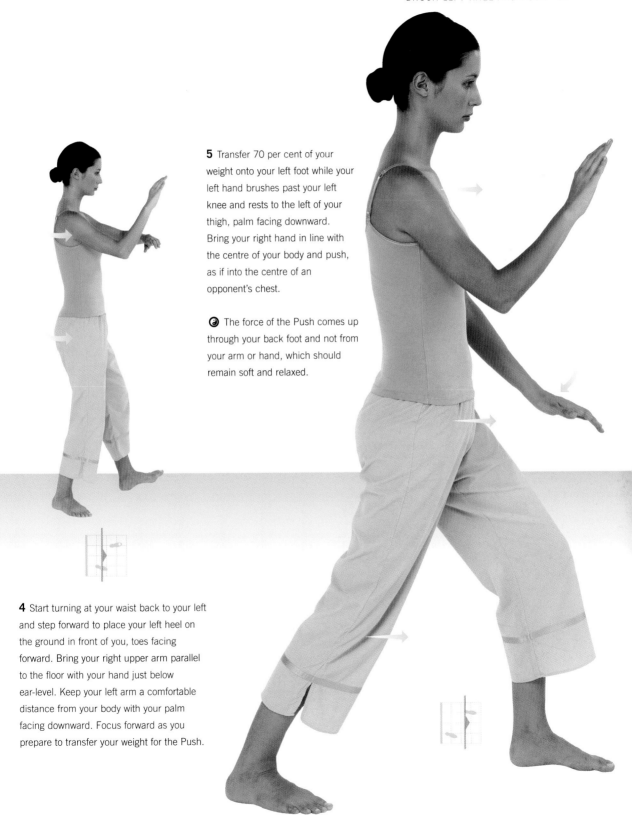

5 Transfer 70 per cent of your weight onto your left foot while your left hand brushes past your left knee and rests to the left of your thigh, palm facing downward. Bring your right hand in line with the centre of your body and push, as if into the centre of an opponent's chest.

☯ The force of the Push comes up through your back foot and not from your arm or hand, which should remain soft and relaxed.

4 Start turning at your waist back to your left and step forward to place your left heel on the ground in front of you, toes facing forward. Bring your right upper arm parallel to the floor with your hand just below ear-level. Keep your left arm a comfortable distance from your body with your palm facing downward. Focus forward as you prepare to transfer your weight for the Push.

step up to play guitar

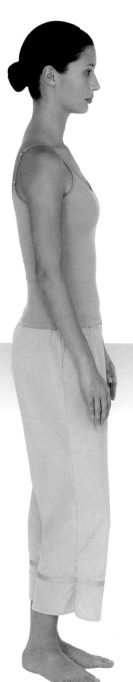

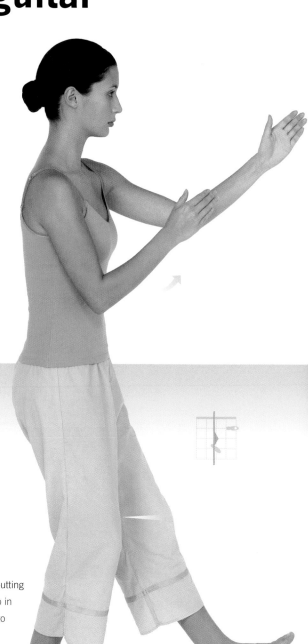

1 Shift all of your weight onto your right foot and then bring your left foot next to it so that you are standing with both feet together. Drop your arms by your sides.

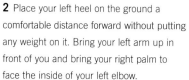

2 Place your left heel on the ground a comfortable distance forward without putting any weight on it. Bring your left arm up in front of you and bring your right palm to face the inside of your left elbow.

brush left knee and push

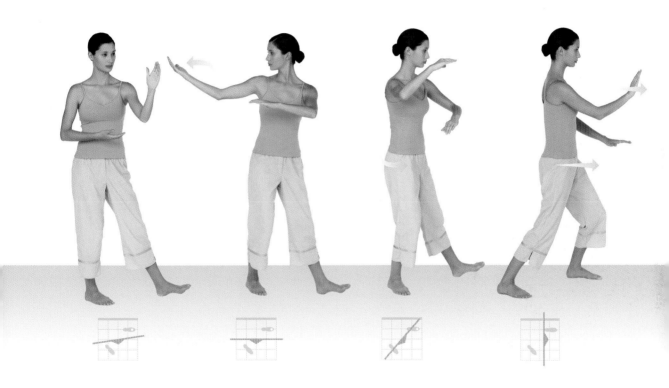

1 Turn from your waist toward your right. Bring your right forearm horizontally in front of your body, palm facing up. Keep a sense of openness under your arms.

2 Extend your right arm to the side, palm facing upward. Bring your left forearm parallel to your body, palm facing down. Turn your head to look over your right shoulder.

3 Turn toward the left. Bend your right arm in front of you at head height, palm facing down. Lower your left arm slightly.

4 Turn to face the left with your right hand in line with the centre of your body, palm facing out. Shift your weight onto your left foot and push into the chest of an imaginary opponent. The force of the Push comes up through your back foot.

step up, parry and punch

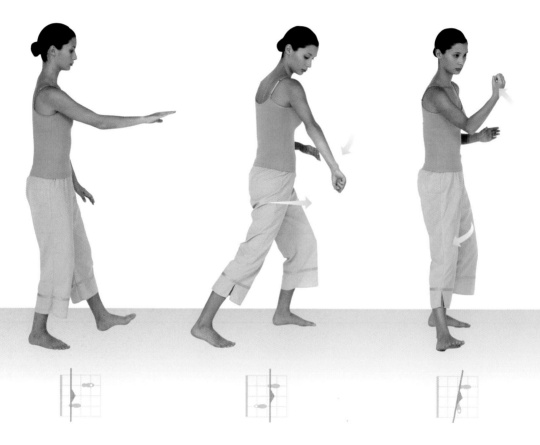

1 Transfer your weight back onto your right foot while turning slightly to your left from your waist. Allow your right arm to lengthen without locking your elbow. Keep your left hand close to your waist, palm facing down.

2 Transfer your weight onto your left foot. Lower your right arm a little and form a soft fist with your right hand. Keep your centre of gravity low and don't straighten your left leg. Keep your shoulders down and a sense of space between your arms and body.

3 Step your right foot forward, toes pointing to the right. Turn from your waist toward the right. Turn your right hand over and raise your fist in front of your face. Take care not to lock your right leg or transfer any weight forward at this point. Move your left hand so that the palm faces the inside of your right elbow.

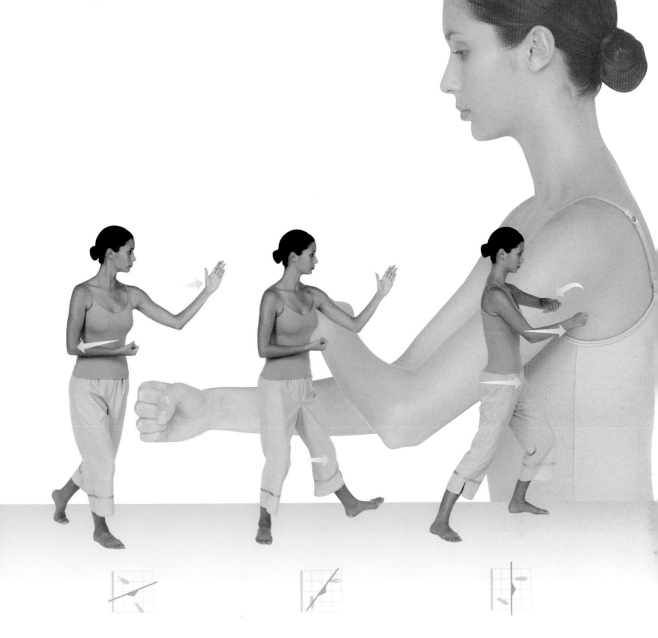

4 Transfer all of your weight onto your right foot and turn from your waist to the right. Allow your left hand to extend in front of you. As you transfer your weight, drop your right hand to your waist with your fist at your side. Keep your right knee bent and don't let your right elbow go behind your body.

5 Step forward with your left foot. Transfer 70 per cent of your weight onto your left foot and turn at your waist toward the left. Let your upper body remain light and open.

6 Square up your body to face forward. Extend the fist of your right hand forward to the centre of your body, a forearm's length in front of you. Bring your left arm across the front of your body, parallel to the floor, palm facing downward.

retract and cross hands

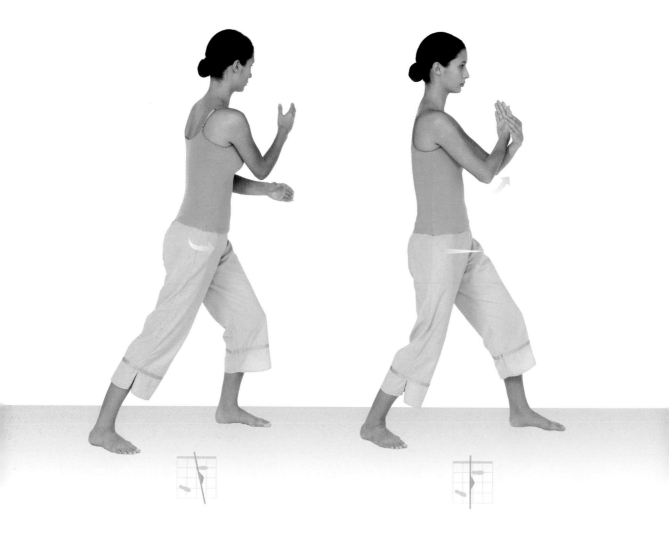

1 Turn from your waist toward the left. As you turn, open your fist and let your right palm face to the left. Bring your left palm under your right elbow. Keep your shoulders down and a sense of openness under your arms.

2 Shift 70 per cent of your weight back onto your right foot. At the same time, bring your left hand up so that it crosses the outside of your right wrist. Keep your arms a good distance from your body and your shoulders relaxed. Don't lean back.

push 1 and 2

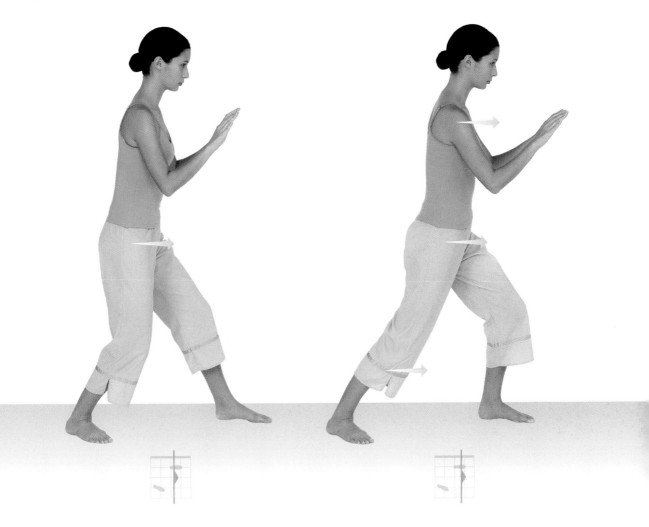

1 Drop your elbows a little more, without bringing them behind your body. Bring your hands in front of your body with your palms facing out ready to push into the centre of an imaginary opponent's chest. Keep your left knee relaxed and not locked.

2 Transfer 70 per cent of your weight forward onto your left foot, but don't let your left knee extend beyond your toes. Keep your arms relaxed and soft as you extend them forward for an uprooting push to a potential opponent. Focus straight ahead.

apparent closure 1 and 2

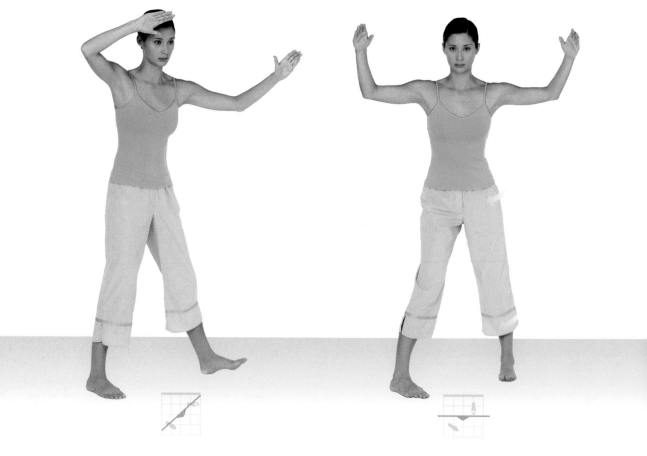

1 Start to shift your weight back onto your right foot while turning on the heel of your left foot. As you turn from your waist to the right, raise your right arm in a circular movement above your head. Do the same with your left arm so that you end up with an open posture, arms extended on either side. Keep your shoulders down and your breath relaxed in your lower abdomen.

☯ The word "apparent" in the title of these postures refers to the fact that this is the end of only the first section of Cheng Man Ching's Short Yang Form.

2 Keep turning at your waist until your body faces forward. Transfer all your weight onto your left foot. Keep your feet shoulder-distance apart.

cross hands and close

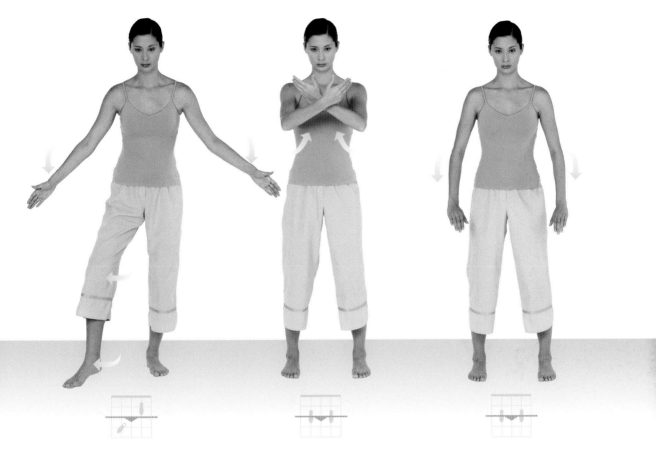

1 Lower your arms on either side of your body. Turn your right foot to point toward the right.

2 Bring your right foot next to your left foot and, with your toes pointing slightly inward, divide your weight equally across each foot. Cross your arms in front of your body, right arm on the outside, palms facing inward. Keep a comfortable space between your arms and your body. Your knees should be soft and your breath relaxed in your lower abdomen.

3 Keep your weight equally divided across both feet and slowly drop your arms to each side. Keep your palms open and relaxed.

checking your postures

Brush Left Knee and Push (side view of step 5, see pages 96–7)

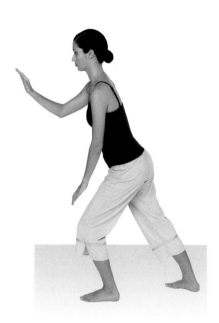 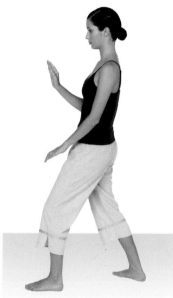 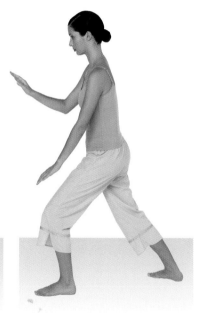

INCORRECT

The student is leaning too far forward here. Her front knee is too far over her toes and her arms are extended too far beyond her body. Her hips are rising and creating an unnatural bend in her back. It is very likely that she will be top-heavy and easily pulled forward, off balance.

INCORRECT

Although the student has most of her weight on her front foot, she is leaning back with her upper body. This means she has a very weak connection with the ground through her front foot. This would result in a highly ineffective Push.

CORRECT

This is the correct way to do the posture. The student's back is in alignment, her hips are tucked in, her front knee is behind her toes and her body is in a good upright position. The power of the Push will come from her connection with the ground through her back foot. This power will travel directly to her hand without being disturbed through misalignment.

When you have become familiar with the postures in this chapter, use the pictures below to check that you are performing them correctly. The most common mistakes that students make are to lean too far forward, backward or to the side. These mistakes can happen in any posture but are particularly common in Brush Left Knee and Push (see pages 96–7 and 99) and Single Whip (see pages 90–91). Try to keep your body in an upright position throughout your practice.

Single Whip (front view, see pages 90–91)

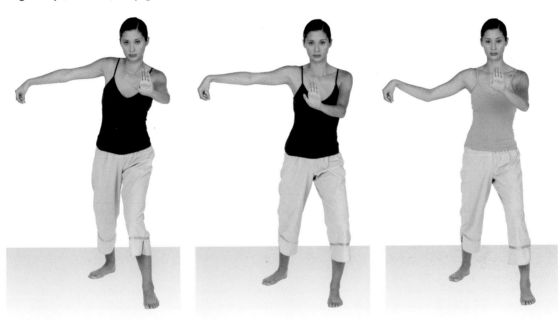

INCORRECT

The student is leaning to the side here and her front knee is folding inward. Because of this instability, her arm has extended too far out to the side in a subconscious effort to aid her balance.

INCORRECT

Here, the student's left arm has crossed too far to the other side of her body rather than staying at the centre line. She is turning too far at her waist instead of facing straight ahead in the direction she is pushing. Her front foot is also turning inward rather than pointing straight forward.

CORRECT

This is the correct way to do the posture. The student's left arm is central to her body; her toes, waist and head are pointing straight ahead; and she is not leaning to one side or the other.

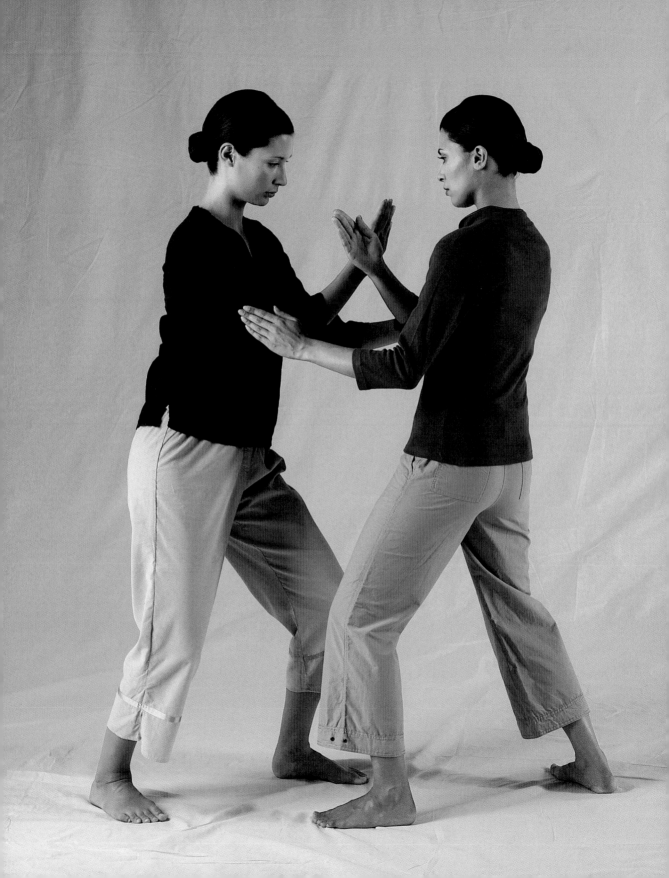

partner exercises

Although most people are familiar with the solo aspects of tai chi, much can be gained through practising with a partner or opponent. In tai chi – as in many other aspects of life – we can learn about ourselves by how we interact with others.

When training with a partner, you need to employ co-operation. If you are too hard or aggressive, your partner may close down, physically, mentally and emotionally. Try to test each other's limitations in a gradual and sensitive way. Get a sense of how you each use your body and how effective your movements are. Working in a spirit of mutual exploration is more creative and productive than one of competition.

yielding to a partner

A basic principle of tai chi is to move in the direction of the energy that is coming toward you. This simple exercise will help you to yield to your partner's energy.

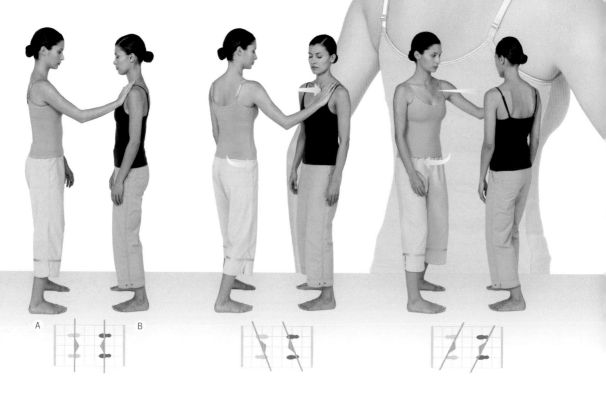

1 Stand opposite each other, roughly an arm's length apart. Both partners should have soft knees and feel connected to the ground. Partner A will push and partner B will yield. Partner A places their right palm softly on B's body, to the left of their upper chest. Take a moment to feel relaxed and connected.

2 Partner A applies gentle but firm pressure by turning toward the left at the waist and pushing their arm "through" B. Partner B moves only as much as is required.

3 Partner A then places their left hand on the right side of B's upper chest. Partner A turns at the waist toward the right and applies firm pressure through B. Again, B moves only as much as is necessary.

When you are both familiar with this exercise, you can try increasing the speed and pressure of the push. The person in the yielding role can also try closing their eyes – the absence of visual information helps you to respond more sensitively to touch.

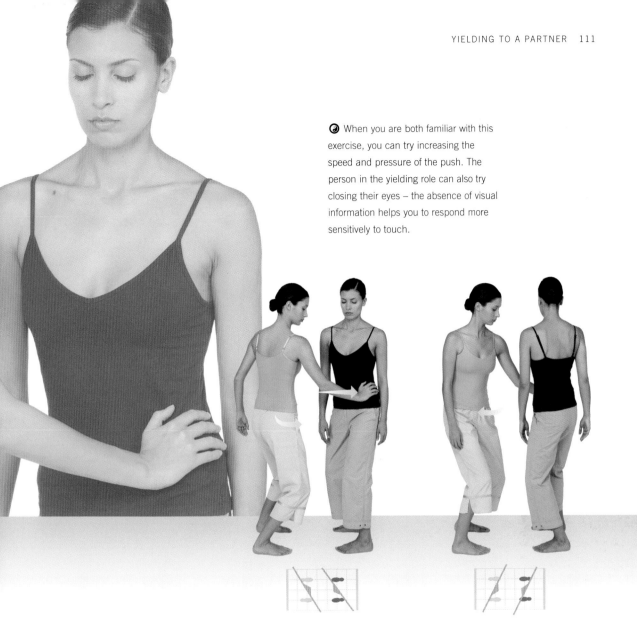

4 Partner A places their right hand on the left side of B's pelvis, then turns to the left and pushes B. Partner B yields as much as is appropriate.

5 Partner A places their left hand on the right side of B's pelvis, then turns to the right and pushes B. Again, B yields as much as is appropriate. Now swap roles.

sticking hands

This exercise helps you to relax, gain confidence and develop sensitivity to a partner's energy. It also teaches you to react quickly and fluidly. Take it in turns to lead each other.

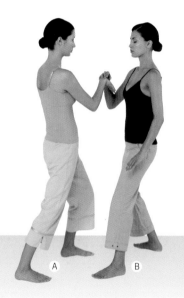

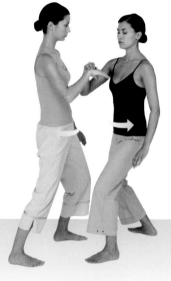

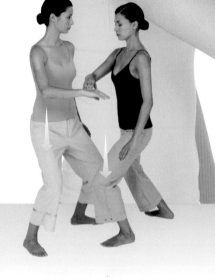

1 Both partners stand facing each other with their left feet forward. Partner B rests their fingers on A's outstretched wrist (right fingers on right wrist or left fingers on left wrist) and closes their eyes. Both partners take a few moments to tune in to each other.

2 Partner A starts to turn slowly to the right from their waist. Partner B keeps their eyes closed and tries to move in synchrony with A.

3 Partner A tries gently to extend B's ability to move in a relaxed, fluid manner by turning more to the right, sinking at the knees and lowering their right arm. Partner B tries to sense where they are being led.

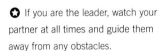

If you are the leader, watch your partner at all times and guide them away from any obstacles.

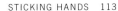

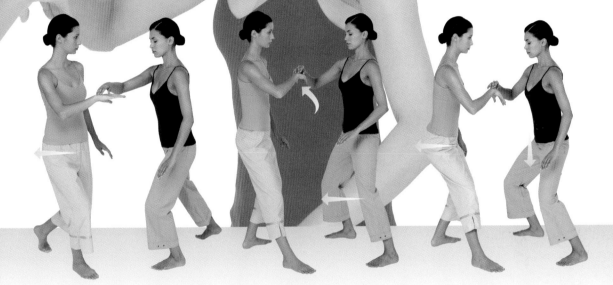

4 Partner A steps back with their left foot and B follows with their body. As both partners move, they should keep their shoulders and elbows down and their arms relaxed rather than fully extended.

5 Partner A shifts their entire weight onto their left foot and turns toward the left. Partner B moves their right foot forward. Both partners should keep their breathing relaxed in the lower abdomen, and the upper body light and open – this makes it easier for B to sense movement.

6 Partner A sinks at their knees and lowers their right arm. Partner B follows. Both partners should begin all of their movements from the waist. The arms shouldn't move independently of the waist.

tui shou – single

Tui Shou means "pushing hands". These exercises are a bridge between the Hand Form and the martial applications of tai chi. They help you to overcome an attack with minimum force.

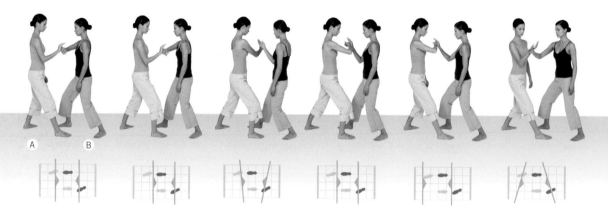

1 Partner A stands facing their partner, right foot facing forward and left foot turned out. The inside of B's right foot is opposite the inside of A's right foot. Partner B raises their arm, wrist opposite the chest. Partner A puts the heel of their hand on the back of B's wrist.

2 Partner A transfers their weight forward, pushing B's hand to the centre of their chest in an attempt to make them lose their balance. Partner B moves their weight back, relative to A's advance.

3 Partner B turns at their waist toward the right and turns their right hand to push away A. Both of you should maintain soft hands during this turn, and turn your palms to face upward just as they reach the limits of their push. The push is now neutralized.

4 Both partners turn at the waist to face each other. Partner B puts the heel of their hand on the front of A's wrist with the intention of pushing forward toward the middle of their chest. Now you have reversed roles.

5 Partner B transfers their weight forward, pushing A's hand to the centre of their chest in an attempt to make them lose their balance. Partner A moves their weight back, relative to B's advance.

6 Partner A turns at their waist toward the right and turns their right hand to push away B. Both partners should maintain soft hands during this turn, and turn their palms to face upward just as they reach the limits of the push. The push is now neutralized.

tui shou – double

This "double hands" version of the previous exercise is great for developing stability, sensitivity and fast reflexes, and the ability to read the intentions of others.

☯ Tune in to how much force is coming toward you. You can neutralize your opponent with a small turn if you can sense where their centre is.

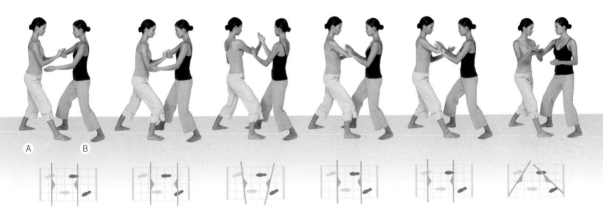

A   B

1 Adopt the same foot positions as for step 1 of Tui Shou – single. Partner B raises their right forearm in front of their chest. Partner A places the heels of both hands on B's arm (at the wrist and just before the elbow). Partner B moves their left hand toward A's elbow.

2 Partner A transfers their weight forward and pushes toward B's chest in an attempt to push them over. Partner B brings their left hand to meet A's elbow.

3 Partner B moves their weight back in relation to A's push, turns at their waist toward the right, and uses their right hand to push away A's right hand. Partner B keeps the palm of the left hand at the outside of A's elbow to create a fulcrum. The push is now neutralized.

4 Both partners turn to face each other and A raises their right forearm in front of their chest. Partner B places the heels of both hands on A's arms. Now you have reversed roles.

5 Partner B transfers their weight forward and pushes their hands forward toward the middle of A's chest in an attempt to push them over. Partner A brings their left hand to meet B's elbow.

6 Partner A moves their weight back in relation to B's push, turns at their waist toward the right, and uses their right hand to push away B's right hand. Partner A keeps the palm of the left hand at the outside of A's elbow to create a fulcrum. The push is now neutralized.

lift hands

This is the first movement in the Hand Form.
Practising this partner version gives you a
sense of how energy flows through your body.

🌀 Don't block or push away your opponent's oncoming force.
Go in the direction of the force, so that as you lift your arms,
you have a sense of drawing their arms in and upward.

Martial Applications

Tai chi was created as a martial art. All of the
postures and linking movements have self-defence
applications. Although these skills may have been
useful in the early days of tai chi, today there is less
need to use your arms and legs to defend yourself.
If you don't want to use tai chi as a martial art, you
can still benefit from practising martial applications
– the exercises in the rest of this chapter will help
you to use your body in a relaxed, focused manner.

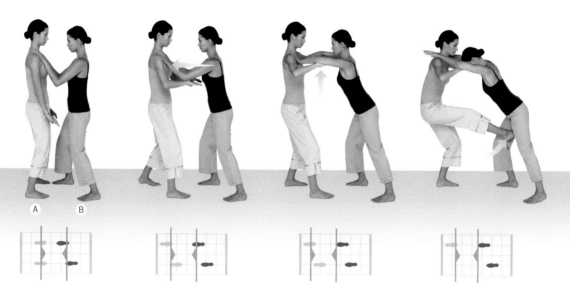

1 Stand facing each other
with your feet shoulder-width
apart. Partner B puts their
hands on A's upper chest,
in preparation to push A over.

2 As B begins to push, A
brings their wrists under B's
elbows. To decrease the
possibility of being pushed
over, A can take a step
backward as the push
comes toward them.

3 Partner A pushes B's arms
up to render the attack
ineffective.

4 Partner A pushes B's arms
over A's shoulders. Then as
B's energy comes toward
them, A raises their right foot
as if they are going to kick
partner B's groin. Now
swap roles.

catch a ball

This is the partner version of the movement that occurs immediately before Prepare to Ward-off in the Hand Form (see page 84). You can do it straight after Lift Hands (opposite).

☯ If you are receiving the attack, keep your arms open and relaxed with your palms facing each other. Keep your upper arm in line with the centre of your chest and your lower arm close to waist height. Don't force your opponent's over-balancing. It is only by connecting to the extreme end of their oncoming force that you can neutralize their attack with minimum force.

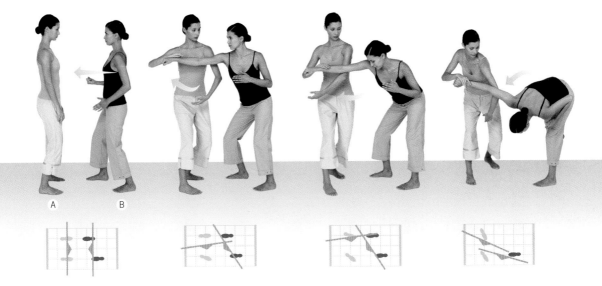

A   B

1 Stand facing each other with your feet shoulder-width apart. Partner B raises their right fist in preparation to punch. Partner B's left hand stays near their waist, palm facing inward.

2 Partner B transfers their weight forward and extends their right arm in a punch. Their left hand is raised to chest height. Partner A turns at the waist toward the right and their right hand makes contact with B's right wrist.

3 As the punch advances, A turns further toward the right at the waist and allows the outside of their left arm to make contact with B's elbow joint.

4 As the punch reaches its extreme point, A continues turning with their arm against partner B's elbow joint – this will pull partner B down and over-balance them. Now swap roles.

roll back 1

Here are some more movements from the Hand Form that you can practise with a partner. They are designed to protect you from an opponent's punch.

☯ Roll Back is most effective as a self-defence technique when your opponent doesn't realize what is happening. Softly lead your opponent's force, slightly ahead of where you sense they want it to go.

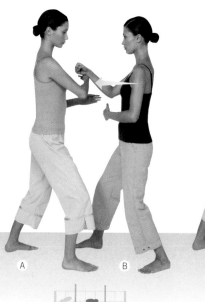
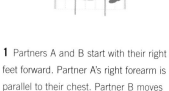

A   B

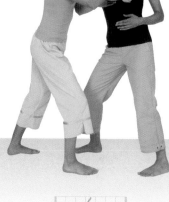

1 Partners A and B start with their right feet forward. Partner A's right forearm is parallel to their chest. Partner B moves their right hand forward in a punch. Partner A meets the punch softly with their right forearm and moves their left hand toward B's right elbow.

2 Partner A shifts their weight forward and turns to the right. They roll their right forearm on top of B's forearm and grasp B's right elbow with their left hand. This takes A's body away from the punch while diverting the attack to the side using minimal force.

3 Partner B retreats as they sense A's oncoming force. Partner A should "stick and follow" by bringing the heel of their right hand under B's chin – this will cause B to lean backward and, ultimately, fall.

roll back 2

☯ Don't resort to using muscular energy and strength. By "sticking" to your opponent's movement, you can overcome their attack with minimal force.

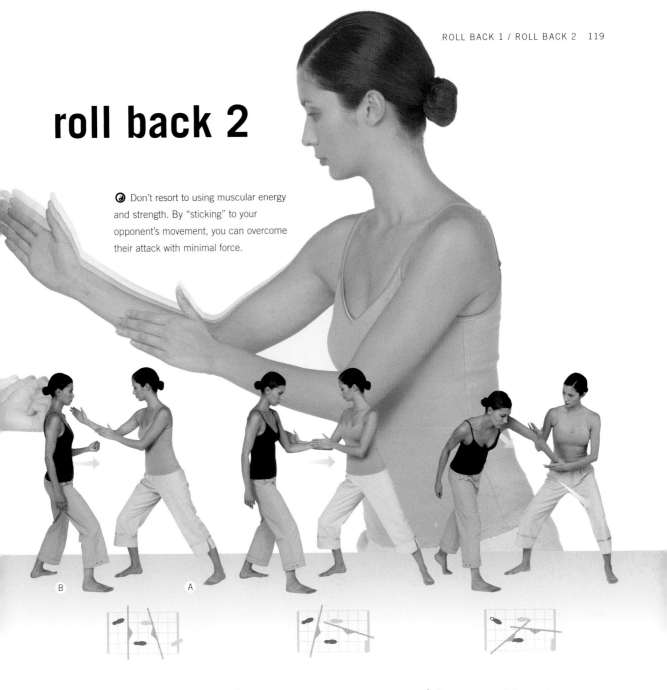

B   A

1 Partner A stands with their weight on their right leg and their arms stretched out in front (but not locked). Their left hand should be opposite their right elbow. Partner B stands with their weight on their left leg and prepares to punch with their left arm.

2 Partner B extends their left arm forward in a punch. Partner A meets the punch by bringing their right hand to contact B's left elbow and their left hand to contact the inside of B's left wrist. Partner A begins to turn to the left.

3 As the force of B's punch comes through, A keeps turning at the waist to the left, maintaining the connection with B's elbow and wrist. This will cause B to over-balance and fall forward.

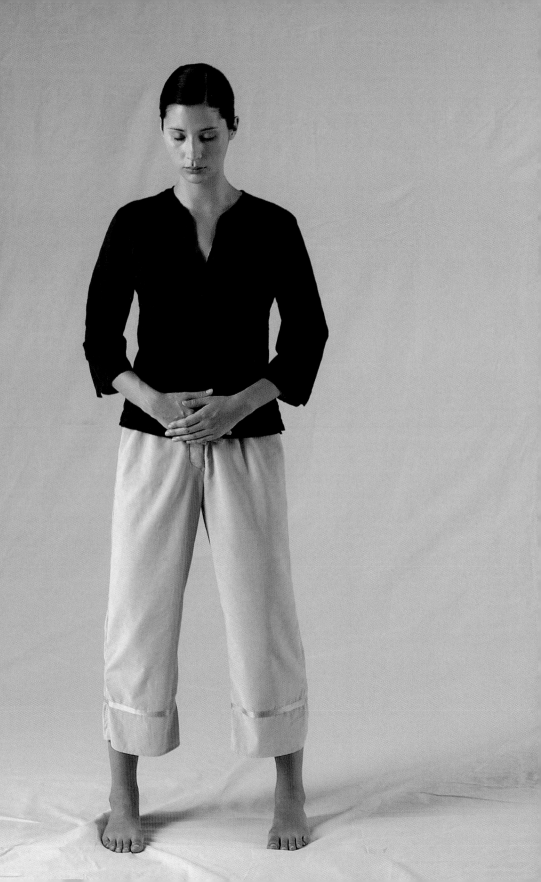

meditation

Meditation is no longer the domain of the dedicated monk or seeker of enlightenment. It is now widely accepted as an effective tool for coping with the stresses of 21st-century living. At today's hectic pace of life, we are frequently taken away from our centre and out of touch with our inner selves – meditation is the key to restoring harmony and balance.

There are many different ways to meditate and it's important to find a style that works for you. Tai chi itself is a form of moving meditation. This chapter explores this aspect of tai chi practice, as well as offering two other meditation exercises – one walking, the other sitting.

tai chi as moving meditation

Tai chi is often referred to as moving meditation. Once you have learned the rudiments of the individual postures and you can do the connecting movements without having to think about them, you start to move in a free-flowing, undisturbed manner. Over time, this frees the mind and you may start to notice that you enter a state of mental stillness when you do tai chi. Ultimately, the goal is to transfer this peaceful state into the rest of your life too.

Being rather than doing

In the early stages of learning you are more likely to be *doing* tai chi rather than *being* tai chi. The difference is that in the first case there is a voice inside your head telling you how to move – and monitoring your performance – and in the second case, you are in a state of pure and mindful flow in which there is simply no need to think. When you get to this level of familiarity, your body will simply move through the postures and you no longer need to consciously think about them. Your knowledge about tai chi has become stored in your body.

When tai chi becomes meditation

How do you know when you have stopped doing, and started being tai chi? You may notice that as you move through the postures you feel a growing sense of calmness and serenity. You may be less aware of the passing of time. You may also observe that your breathing is naturally relaxed and you have a sense of oneness with your environment. Rather than thinking about the technicalities of the movements, you are just flowing smoothly through space, and the air passes slowly around your body as you move from one posture to the next. All or any of these observations mean that you are entering a meditative state during your tai chi practice. Your movements connect you with something else other than space and time. As the shapes you make with your body subtly change the landscape, you start to feel that you are joined to the greater collective consciousness.

Blocks to meditation

The primary objective in most systems of meditation is to calm the mind. This is also known as "taming the tiger". The biggest block to achieving a meditative state is to have a busy mind; to be constantly preoccupied with thoughts. If you find that you are distracted during your tai chi practice, it's especially important to create some time beforehand in which you allow yourself quietly to unwind. You can do this by practising some chi kung exercises or just by sitting still in a calm environment.

Unsteady transitions can also act as a block to meditation. Transitions are the movements that connect one posture to another to create a smooth and flowing sequence in tai chi (see pages 78–79). It's common for students of tai chi to work hard on the individual postures but to neglect the transitions. So, even if you do a posture perfectly, an unsteady transition will disturb your mental stillness and equilibrium. As you practise tai chi, pay close attention to any transitions that are unsteady and repeat them until you can do them with ease.

Using your imagination

You can help yourself to get into a meditative state by identifying with the spirit of the creatures whose characteristics informed the creation of tai chi. Try imagining that you are a tiger or crane as you practise the Hand Form. See how this affects your performance. You may discover aspects of your character that you were previously unaware of!

Applying meditation to your life

Tai chi is a holistic process that integrates your mind, body and spirit. Reaching a calm, centred, meditative state in your daily tai chi practice is just the first step – your ultimate goal is to carry this state into all aspects of your daily life. The more you practise tai chi, the more you will become aware of how you relate to others and how your body is affected in times of stress. This increased awareness will allow you to take steps to calm yourself quickly whenever your equilibrium is disturbed. If you are able to connect to your breath in your lower abdomen, it is very unlikely that you will become upset in response to anger or upset in others. You will also become increasingly aware of how quickly anger rises in others. Through discovering a greater sense of yourself through the meditative process of tai chi you will help to cultivate a sense of calmness in all your relationships. But don't expect to immediately change into a perfect human being – such a thing doesn't exist. Neither do perfect relationships. Just be happier in the knowledge that you are more sensitive to the times when you "come out of yourself" and that you know how to restore yourself to a state of equanimity.

BELOW: As you move through the postures of tai chi, try to get a sense of groundedness and flow. Imagine how corn blows and bends in the wind yet is firmly rooted in the ground.

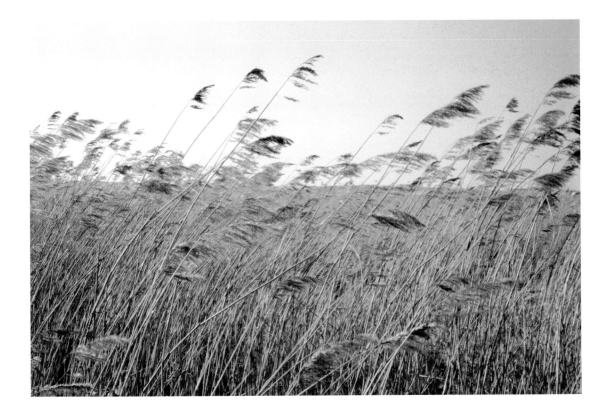

inner awareness during tai chi

The journey of tai chi takes you from the external – in which your focus is on the positioning and movements of your body – to the internal. When you get to the point at which you can do the postures with ease, you can start to concentrate on the subtleties of tai chi. This concentration takes you on a path to meditation.

Every student has to go through a learning curve in tai chi. Your first job is to become familiar with the shapes of the postures and how to move from one to another in a smooth and flowing way. This takes a great deal of practice and, unfortunately, the strong focus on the external can sometimes have the effect of divorcing you from your inner self. The real work of tai chi comes much later when you are able to stop thinking about the movements and patterns of your body and start to turn your attention inward. Ultimately, tai chi is about self-discovery and self-development. Once you are able to apply an inner focus during your practice, you are opening the door to a meditative state of mind and all the benefits that this brings.

Turning your attention inward

Entering a meditative state of mind is not a skill that you can learn directly by following a set sequence of steps. Instead, you can try to cultivate the circumstances that are conducive to meditation. For example, you can focus on what is happening inside your body when you practise the Hand Form.

The first sense of inner awareness begins with the Beginning Posture (see page 80) in which you simply stand still. Try to listen to what is happening within your body. Become aware of any little areas of discomfort. Try making minute adjustments to your posture with the aim of finding the best way of supporting your skeleton with the minimum of physical tension.

As you move from the Beginning Posture to the other postures of the Form, pay attention to your hands, fingers, arms and shoulders and try to keep them relaxed. A common mistake

that students make is to keep their shoulders and arms relaxed while their fingers are as stiff as rods! Your teacher will easily notice these things and can point them out to you, but far better is to cultivate your own awareness of the signs of stress in your body. As you progress through the Hand Form, keep your attention focused on the internal aspects of each posture and movement. How does it feel when you transfer your weight from one foot to the next? How does it feel to raise one arm and drop the other? What happens inside your body when you sink down and rise up again? What happens to your breath when you inhale? How deep and smooth is your breathing? All of these observations will further your knowledge of yourself.

Every practice is different

When you do tai chi, accept that each practice will be different. Sometimes you will be able to turn your attention inward in the way I've described. At other times you may find that you need to go back to focusing on the external aspects of the postures. Often – or even most of the time – you may have a voice inside your head that says, "Oops! I nearly stumbled there", or "Ouch, my knee hurt a little that time." The important thing is to acknowledge this without being distracted by it. Don't be put off if you think you've practised badly – let the critical voice in your head come and go. Accept that you will make errors and move on from them.

OPPOSITE: This apparently simple posture can be deeply meditative. Once your body has settled into a comfortable standing position you can focus on your internal state.

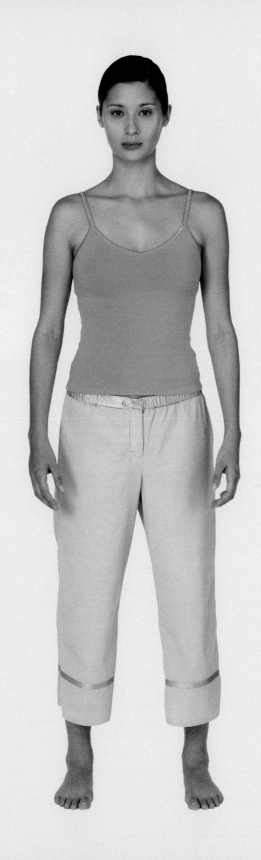

inner awareness during partner work

Solo tai chi practice is an excellent way to learn about your relationship with yourself, but if you want to learn how you relate to others, doing tai chi with a partner can reveal a great deal. In time, it can also help you to cultivate mental stillness when you are in conflict with others.

If you have been trying to develop your inner awareness during your solo tai chi practice, your next challenge is to apply this awareness during partner work. This is more difficult – when an opponent is trying to unbalance you or push you over, your first response is likely to be escape or retaliation. Over time you can train yourself to focus on the internal instead of the external so that you can monitor your reactions to attack, both physical and psychological. The next step is to greet attack with softness and yielding rather than tension or aggression. Getting into this inwardly-focused, meditative state of mind will serve you well, not just in tai chi, but in the rest of your life too.

Once you are familiar with the techniques of the following three exercises, try practising them with an inward focus.

Sticking Hands

The Sticking Hands exercise (see pages 112–13) is one step beyond the solo practice of tai chi. It is like doing the Hand Form while someone is attempting to unbalance you slightly. This can be likened to a minor disagreement between friends. As you do the exercise, ask yourself whether you find it easy or difficult to recover your centre and stay relaxed? Observe when you feel comfortable and relaxed, and when you feel challenged. Perhaps your partner moved more quickly than you wanted them to or maybe there were times when you felt you couldn't keep your fingers in contact with their wrist? By applying this inner awareness you will develop a clearer sense of what is required for you to stay stable and relaxed when under slight pressure.

Tui Shou – single

In Tui Shou – single (see page 114) you and your partner are starting to get a little more serious! Instead of leading you safely around the room, your partner is actually trying to push you over, albeit in a gentle, controlled way. In a real-life setting, this is like someone getting close to the truth in an argument. They've touched a raw nerve. Observe your reactions to this. When they are pushing toward your centre, trying to over-balance you, do you stay cool and relaxed, or do you start to tense up? It is only by developing your inner awareness that you begin to understand how you react under pressure. Once you have this understanding, you can change your reactions and function more effectively.

Tui Shou – double

In Tui Shou – double (see page 115) the push is more direct and it is harder to get out of. This is like getting cornered by your boss when they discover you haven't done your work – you're stuck and the pressure keeps coming. Observe your reaction to this exercise. Notice whether your shoulders rise up, and whether you begin to sweat or show any other signs of nervous tension. Double-hand pushing can help you develop a very clear sense of how you react and at what point you get stuck when you're under extreme pressure.

OPPOSITE: Practising tai chi exercises with a partner encourages you to stay centred and focused. It also increases your sensitivity to the energy of others.

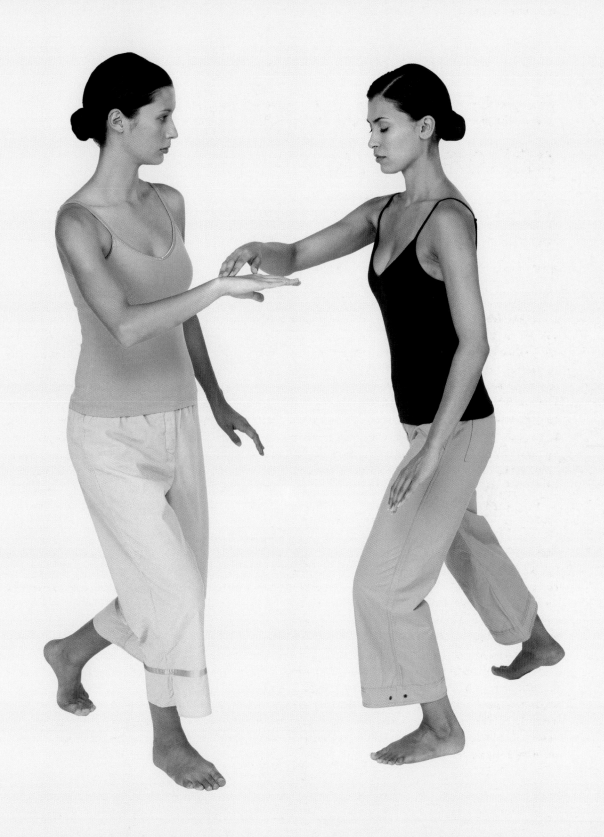

walking meditation

There are many varieties of walking meditation – you can vary the position of your arms, breathe in time with your steps and you can even walk backward. This exercise is one of the simplest which, for me, makes it all-the-more valuable. The more tai chi or chi kung you do, the more you will begin to appreciate that it is often the most basic exercises, constantly repeated, that deepen your understanding and development.

1 Start by standing with your feet shoulder-distance apart and your weight evenly distributed between both feet. Soften your knees and get a sense of being connected to the earth through the Yongquan points (see page 26) on the soles of your feet (behind the ball, in the centre). It may help to imagine roots growing from this point into the ground beneath you. When you feel connected downward, allow your breath to settle in your lower abdomen. Place your palms gently against your stomach at the area of the lower dantien (see page 27) or gently clasp your hands at abdomen-level, palms facing upward. Take a few moments to establish your connection with the earth. Check that your knees are not dropping inward, relax your shoulders, and imagine your head is lightly suspended from above.

2 With a natural and comfortable step, place your left heel gently on the ground in front of you. Slowly transfer your weight onto that foot as if you are testing to see whether the ground can take you. Continue until more of your foot comes in contact with the earth and is flat on the ground. Bring all of your weight onto this foot and establish a firm connection with the earth.

3 Bring your right heel off the ground so that just your toes are in contact with the ground. Bend the knee of your left leg.

4 Lift your right toes off the ground and bring your right foot forward past your left foot.

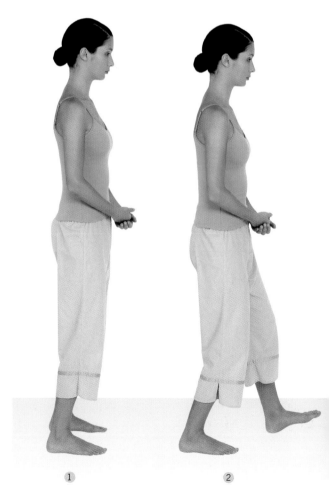

1   2

5 Gently place the heel of your right foot on the ground in front of your left foot. Once again, imagine that you are testing to see whether the ground can support your weight.

6 Slowly lower the whole of your right foot onto the ground and transfer your weight onto it. Keep doing this slow, conscious stepping and be mindful of each act of weight transference from one foot to another. Think about how your feet are connected with the earth and how your head is open to the heavens. Keep your breathing slow and soft in your lower dantien. Don't raise your knees too high. If you begin to shake, lose your balance or you become distracted, just bring your attention back to your

breathing. Remaining quietly focused on your breath will help your stance to stay stable and strong.

Moving your arms with your body

You can vary this exercise by allowing your arms to move with your body. Start with your arms at your sides with your palms softly open and facing downward, as if you are warming them at a fire. Then, as you step forward, allow your arms to rise slowly by your sides. Keep them soft and open. When your front foot is fully in contact with the ground and you are beginning to transfer your weight forward, allow your arms gently to come back down to rest by your sides.

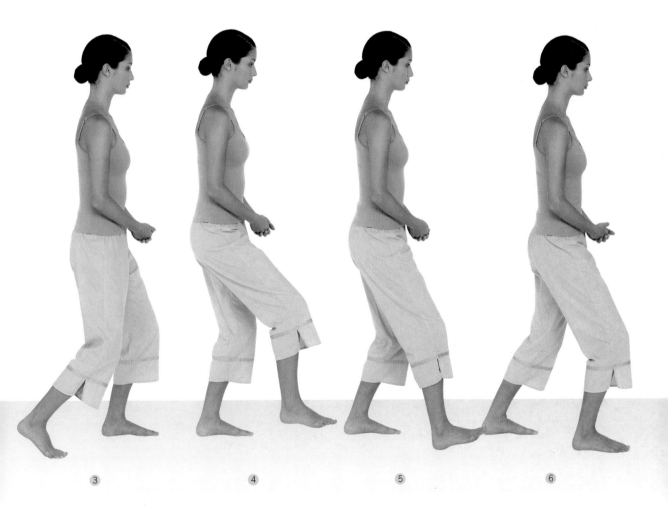

③   ④   ⑤   ⑥

sitting meditation

This sitting meditation promotes the flow of chi (energy) around your body and increases your sense of vitality. It's a particularly good meditation to try if you are feeling weak or fatigued, or if you have limited mobility.

1 Find a place where you can sit comfortably and quietly by yourself, where you won't be disturbed by ringing telephones or any other external noises. If possible, choose a place in which there is a flow of fresh, clean air, rather than artificial ventilation or central heating.

2 Place a chair in your chosen space and sit down. Softly close your eyes. Bring your attention to your breathing and notice which parts of your body are moving because of the in and out flow of your breath. Slowly allow your breathing to settle in your lower abdomen.

3 Get a sense of how you are sitting in the chair. Which parts of your body are most in contact with the chair? Try to feel connected to the chair through your sitting bones rather than through your back. Imagine that your head is like a balloon floating up in the air. Allow your spine to lengthen and open. Let your shoulders drop and your chest relax inward a little. Connect the tip of your tongue to the roof of your mouth, just behind your upper front teeth. This position will allow your body's internal energy to move comfortably through your meridians.

4 Bring your attention to your feet. At the centre of the soles of your feet is the Yongquan point – this is where you draw up energy from the earth. Imagine energy entering your feet at this point and travelling through your feet to your heels and then your ankle joints. Get a sense of the shape of your feet in your shoes and think about them relaxing and taking up a little more surface area. Let your ankle joints loosen as the energy begins

to travel up the insides of your calves to your knee joints. Focus on your knee joints for a few moments. Imagine them being looser and more relaxed, perhaps getting a little warmer as the energy passes through them.

5 Let the energy flow upward from the earth through your knee joints and through the insides of your thighs. Imagine two rivers of warm light travelling through your legs in a clear, flowing path and connecting at the base of your spine. Now let the chi travel up inside your spine, through your neck, to a point on the crown of your head known as the Beihui point (see page 26). From here, the energy moves down through the front of your head to where your tongue is in contact with your upper palate, just behind your upper front teeth. Imagine that you are swallowing the energy so that it travels down the front of your body and flows into your lower abdomen (the dantien; see page 27). This is where energy is stored and accumulated.

6 Keep sitting in an open, comfortable way visualizing the flow of energy from the earth, entering your feet and legs and circulating through your body. Imagine how this meditation will help you to clear your meridians, increase your energy flow, and build a store of energy that will sustain you. At the end of your meditation, open your eyes and reconnect with your environment before carrying on with your day.

◉ As you are following the energy around your body, occasionally bring your attention back to your feet and remind yourself of your connection to the earth.

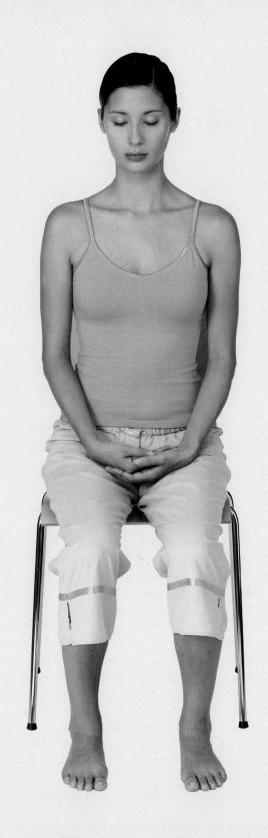

conclusion

Now that you have studied and practised the exercises and postures in chapters 3 to 6, you'd probably like to have an idea of how your tai chi training is developing. One of the hardest things for tai chi students is to evaluate their stages of development in training. There is no tradition of awarding grades or coloured belts (although some schools are now trying to introduce this), so unless you enter competitions, your progress level is not always recognizable.

Although the majority of tai chi practitioners have no interest in taking part in competitions, you can still use competition criteria to assess your training. On page 137, I have included a chart that lists the names of the key movements of the Hand Form together with the criteria on which you would be assessed on in a competition. I issue these sheets to my students so they can use them as personal feedback forms. By knowing the criteria that

judges use in the context of a competition, you will be closer to understanding what makes good tai chi practice. The chart will prompt you to check your posture, martial spirit, degree of relaxation and many other aspects of the art. Don't take self-assessment too seriously – you won't win any prizes by checking your own performance, but you will start to consider all of the different attributes that can inform your practice.

Why are you doing tai chi?

Once you have carefully considered the various attributes of good tai chi practice and found a way regularly to check your development, it's a good time to go back to the starting point. Think about what it was that attracted you to this art. Was it to gain a sense of relaxation and inner peace? Was it to attain a sense of oneness with everything that is going around you? Was it to find a place of calmness that refreshes and invigorates you? Or were you interested in tai chi as a martial art? Whatever your reasons are, they are for you and you alone. By reminding yourself of the reasons why you were interested in tai chi, you will be inspired to continue with the work of practising regularly. Through a quiet, sustained commitment you can get closer to achieving your original goals.

Varying your training pattern

In the early stages of learning tai chi you will spend most of your time trying to get a sense of the shape and form of the individual postures. You will be looking at the pictures in this book, checking that you are in the right position and then trying to make all the postures link up. Obviously this process takes some time. Ultimately, you are looking for a way to repeat the sequences without having continually to consult the images and copy them. One technique for speeding up your learning is to vary your training routine. Here are some suggestions about how to do this:

1. Pick one movement and repeat it. Go over it again and again, paying great attention to your stance and posture. Keep checking the position of your feet. Look at the photographs in this book and re-read the text several times. Work hard to be as accurate as possible.

2. On another occasion, practise a series of postures in a loose manner without worrying if they are correct. Try to get the sequence of movements into your "bodymind" so that it stays there and you are able to repeat it without thinking about what you are doing. Although you may not achieve precision in the individual postures in this way, you will be able to master the order of the postures and how they link together.

3. A third way of practising is to perform a few movements while turning your attention inward. Tune in to your body and breath. Get a deep sense of your balance and your ability to gently place one foot on the ground. Take as long as you like to transfer your weight from one leg to the other. Tuning into your inner self on a regular basis is one of the treasures of tai chi practice. Every time you perform a sequence it will feel different. Just as your emotions shift all the time, so too will the feelings you experience while practising tai chi. It is the ability to listen to ourselves that ultimately informs us of who we really are.

4. As an alternative to connecting with yourself, try connecting with your surroundings. Practising outdoors is by far the best way to get the most from tai chi. Now that most people are familiar with the art, you are less likely to attract attention by practising in public places such as parks. Find a place near some trees or water and take a few minutes to get a sense of the beauty of nature. Connect yourself to the earth and its bounty, enjoy the colours around you, get a sense of the air quality and feel the gentle breeze of the wind on your skin. As you practise tai chi, get a sense of yourself merging with nature and becoming part of the scenery. Practising tai chi in nature can be especially valuable if you live in a city. Stressful city-living increasingly takes us away from all the rejuvenating qualities that can be found outdoors.

Using imagery

Try to set aside a time every day, in a place that makes you feel quiet and comfortable, and practise just for the sake of practice. You can, from time to time, bring new ideas into your training. Go back to Chapter 6 and read through the ways in which you can make your tai chi practice more meditative. For example, think about the animal movements that inspired the beautifully, flowing movements of tai chi. Play around by adopting the various attributes of different creatures – one day you can focus on moving like a snake and the next you can adopt the nature of a strong, lithe tiger. These images will improve your sense of freedom and flow.

Checking on your inner development

Although tai chi is predominantly a physical exercise, it is not merely about performing a routine in an efficient manner with good posture and smooth connections between the sequences. A large part of tai chi work is developing harmony between the body, mind and spirit. You will find that your practice will change not only your posture and the way you move but also your emotions and how you relate to others. Through regular training you will become more focused, calmer and more able to understand or foresee the times when you are getting disturbed, raising your chi, and close to coming out of your centre. By developing a closer connection with your body and your breath, you will be better equipped to calm yourself in times of conflict, to understand and respect the views of others and to maintain a stronger sense of conviction in your beliefs. You will see the danger signs in others when they become over-excited and you will develop the grace to allow them to express their fears or anger without becoming deeply affected by it. Consider the basic principles of the work, the constant interchange of the energies from yin/yang and yang/yin. As Lao Tzu said: "There is nothing as constant as change." It is by observing and adapting to changes that we become more at peace with ourselves and others. When a force comes toward you (yang), whether physical, intellectual or emotional, try to greet it with softness (yin), while remaining calm with a strong sense of inner strength.

Enjoying your practice

Every time you begin the journey of tai chi, find a place of quietness inside yourself as you prepare to experience the sensual pleasure of moving gracefully through the air. Become part of the landscape and merge blissfully with all that is around you without losing sight of your relationship to your inner self and how it connects to everything else. Become part of the bigger picture and discover the joy of being at home inside of yourself. Approach each and every practice session with this potential behind you, and all you were searching for when you picked up this book will become yours.

reflecting on your practice

As I mentioned on page 132, this part of the book is to help you reflect on your tai chi practice and evaluate your development. It should not prompt you to be self-critical! You can copy the chart opposite and use it to record how you think you're progressing, or you can ask your teacher to evaluate you. The 11 aspects of good tai chi practice are as follows:

1. Correct posture: This means that all the different parts of your body are in the right place. Check your posture against the photographs in Chapter 4. Make sure that you feel "connected" and relaxed.

2. Correct stance: Check that your feet are in the right place and your weight is distributed correctly. Refer to the grids underneath the photographs in Chapter 4.

3. Direction: Make sure you are facing the right way. If you practice in the same place on a regular basis, you will become familiar with where you should be facing.

4. Distinguishing yin and yang: In the early stages, this aspect of your training is difficult to achieve. Only through working with a teacher will you really understand yin and yang fully. In the meantime, try to work on the idea of double-weightedness. This means that you carry different amounts of weight in each leg during your tai chi practice. Distributing your weight equally across your legs (except where you are instructed to do so) shows a lack of differentiation between yin and yang.

5. Coordination: Your upper and lower body should move in harmony – each part should move in perfect coordination with the other.

6. Smooth transition: This means moving smoothly from one posture to another. Take the time to slowly transfer your weight from one foot to the next. Ultimately, you should be able to perform the tai chi sequence with no "joins" showing.

7. Intent and focus: When you are clear about how to move through each posture, it should start to look like you really "mean it" when you are practising. To achieve this, you need to focus your mind on each movement before you do it.

8. Balanced turning and stepping: When you stand on one leg, you should be steady, and feel able to take as long as you like before bringing your other foot into contact with the ground. You should be able to place your heel on the ground first and then slowly transfer your weight.

9. Relaxation and softness: All parts of your body (and mind) should be completely relaxed and soft. From time to time, try checking the tendons on the backs of your hands to see if they are fully relaxed.

10. Aesthetic appearance: Simply speaking, your Form should look good. If you are taking part in a competition, the style of your dress and appearance can increase your points in this category, but so too can the style of your performance. When your family and friends begin to feel relaxed while they watch you, then you're probably getting closer to this aspect of good practice.

11. Martial spirit: Of all the attributes, martial spirit is probably one of the hardest to judge. Try to think of all the people in your life who have a certain presence. There is something about them that engages you and makes you interested – this is the quality that you are aiming for. Someone has practised tai chi regularly and who understands the purpose of each posture is most likely to express this martial spirit.

A note for beginners: Don't worry about trying to integrate all of the above aspects of good tai chi practice into your training straight away. Instead give priority to these three aspects, in this order:

1. Correct stance: Concentrate on getting your feet in the right place – this will make you feel more relaxed and comfortable and the transitions from one posture to the next will be easier.

2. Correct posture: Take the time to understand the shape and form of each position. Correct posture makes the work of stepping from one position to the next much easier.

3. Relaxation and softness: Keep this at the back of your mind all the time. By being relaxed and soft you will learn everything much quicker – and you will also feel the benefits of being tension-free!

	CP*	CS	D	Y/Y	Co.	ST	I/F	BTS	R/S	AA	MS
KEY POSTURES											
Beginning											
Lift Hands											
Ward-Off Left											
Ward-Off Right											
Roll Back											
Press											
Push											
Single Whip											
Play Guitar											
Shoulder Stroke											
White Crane Spreads Wings											
Brush Left Knee and Push											
Play Guitar											
Brush Left Knee and Push											
Step Up Parry and Punch											
Push											
Cross Hands											

Student's name:

Period of study:

Date of feedback:

Comments:

* Key to abbreviations

CP: correct posture

CS: correct stance

D: direction

Y/Y: distinguishing yin and yang

Co.: coordination

ST: smooth transition

I/F: intent and focus

BTS: balanced turning and stepping

R/S: relaxation and softness

AA: aesthetic appearance

MS: martial spirit

tai chi organizations

UK

The Tai Chi Union for Great Britain

1 Littlemill Drive

Crookston

Glasgow G53 7GF

Tel: 0141 810 3482

www.taichiunion.com

promo@taichiunion.com

The British Council for Chinese Martial Arts

c/o 110 Frensham Drive

Stockingford

Nuneaton

Warwickshire

CV10 9QL

Tel: 01247 639 4642

www.bccma.com

Tai Chi Caledonia

18 Branziert Road North

Killearn

Stirlingshire

G63 9RF

Tel: 01360 550461

www.taichicaledonia.com

enquiries@taichicaledonia.com

EUROPE

Wudang Tai Chi Chuan

9 Ashfield Road

London N14 7LA

Tel: 020 8368 6815

www.taichichuan.co.uk

The Taijiquan and Qigong Federation for Europe

1 Littlemill Drive

Crookston

Glasgow G53 7GF

Tel: 0141 810 3482

www.tcfe.org

info@tcfe.org

Fédération de Tai Chi Chuan Chi Gong (FTCCG)

17 rue du Louvre

75001 Paris

Tel: +33 1 40 26 95 50

Fax: +33 1 40 26 95 44

ftccg@wanadoo.fr

www.fed-taichichuan.asso.fr

IQTO

Hofgrabengasse 3/13

2490 Ebenfurth

Austria

Tel: +43 (0)664-420 7550

buero@iqtoe.at

www.iqtoe.at

Bulgarian Wushu Federation

Tsar Osvododitel Blvd 25

Sofia 1504

Tel: +359-2-9442337

tradytj@yahoo.com

Taijiquan & Qigong Netzwerk Deutschland

Oberkleener Str. 23

35510 Butzbac

Germany

Tel: +49 511 - 1691767

Fax: +49 511 - 2358536

info@taijiquan-qigong.de

www.taijiquan-qigong.de

Stichting Taijiquan Nederland

Postbus 13264

3507 LG Utrecht

Netherlands

Tel: +31 (0) 30 272 1002

Fax: +31 (0) 30 272 1002

info@taijiquan.nl

www.taijiquan.nl

Paul Silfverstråle

Gustav Adolfsgatan 4

582 20 Linköping

Sweden

Tel: +46 708 939 176

paul@wudang.se

www.wudang.se/stqa/

USA

The National Qigong Association of America

PO Box 270065

St Paul

MN 55127

USA

Tel: (888) 815-1893

www.nqa.org

books and other resources

BIBLIOGRAPHY

Docherty, Dan **Complete Tai Chi Chuan**
(The Crowood Press Ltd, USA, 1997)

Jou Tsung Hwa **The Tao of Tai Chi Chuan**
(Charles E Tuttle, USA, 1980)

A Taoist Classic – The Book of Lao Zi
(Foreign Languages Press, Beijing, 1993)

FURTHER INFORMATION

BOOKS
Cheng Man-ch'ing and Smith, Robert **Tai-Chi**
(Charles E Tuttle, USA, 1967)

Essence of Tai Chi Chuan – The Literary Tradition
(North Atlantic Books, USA, 1979)

Xie Shoude **Competition Routines for Four Styles Taijiquan**
(People's Sports Publishing House, China, 1991)

Docherty, Dan **Instant Tao**
(Red Cinnabar, UK, 1995)

Master Lam Kam-Chuen, **Everyday Chi Kung**
(HarperCollins, USA, 2004)

Jahnke, Roger **The Healing Promise of Qi**
(Contemporary Books, USA & UK, 2002)

Jarmey, Chris **Taiji Qigong**
(Corpus Publishing, USA, 2001)

MacRitchie, James **Chi Kung – Energy for Life**
(Thorsons, USA, 2002)

MAGAZINES
Tai Chi Chuan & Internal Arts (UK)
www.taichiunion.com/magazine.html

European Internal Arts Journal
www.internalartsjournal.com

T'ai Chi Magazine (US)
www.tai-chi.com

DVDS
Tai Chi Short Form – Ronnie Robinson
Beckmann Visual Publishing BDV062

The Chi Kung Way – Ronnie Robinson
Beckmann Visual Publishing BDV061

AUDIO CD
The Tai Chi Classics
Dan Docherty – Luce Condamine
RC Enterprises (www.taichichuan.co.uk)

index

acknowledgments

Picture acknowledgments:

The publisher would like to thank the following people, museums, and photographic libraries for permission to reproduce their material. Every care has been taken to trace copyright holders. However, if we have omitted anyone we apologize and will, if informed, make corrections to any future edition.

Page 15 Yann Layma/Getty Images; 19 PanoramaStock/ Robert Harding World Imagery; 20 Private Collection; 22 Leland Bobbé/Corbis; 25 Tony Waltham/Robert Harding World Imagery; 31 Stuart Mcclymont/Getty; 37 Theo Allofs/Getty Images; 41 Ted Mead/Getty Images; 43 David Paterson/Getty Images; 45 John Henley/Corbis; 46 Robert Llewellyn/Corbis; 123 Plainpicture/Alamy.

Models:

Jasmine Hemsley
Sheri Staplehurst
(from MOT MODELS agency)

Make-up artist:

Jo Jenkins

Ronnie Robinson can be contacted at:

www.chirontaichi.co.uk
secretary@taichiunion.com